# RISING TOGETHER

Rising Together: A Family's Journey
Through Rare Disease and Resilience

Shae Freeman

**Community Responders LLC**

# CONTENTS

Times

# INTRODUCTION:
## *A JOURNEY OF LOVE, STRENGTH, AND HOPE*

As a mother of a child born with a rare disease, I have spent the last 24 years navigating a path that, at times, felt overwhelmingly difficult yet profoundly meaningful. This book is not just a compilation of research and advice—it's a personal reflection of my own experiences, struggles, and triumphs as a parent. From the moment I received the diagnosis that changed my life, I knew that I had been thrust into a world that few people truly understand. And yet, within that world, I found an incredible well of strength, hope, and resilience—qualities that I know you have within you, too.

The road ahead is not easy, and I won't pretend that every day will be filled with victories. But what I can offer you is encouragement: You are not alone. The experiences shared in this book come from a place of deep understanding, having lived through the sleepless nights, the medical appointments, the endless advocacy, and the moments of doubt. It's my hope that through sharing my journey —and the journeys of other parents and caregivers like us—you will find solace, encouragement, and practical tools to help you navigate your own path with your child.

**The Early Days: Finding Strength When You Feel Powerless**
When I first learned of my child's condition, I was overwhelmed with fear and uncertainty. I remember sitting in that sterile doctor's office, hearing words that seemed too big to understand

and wondering how my life would ever be the same. I felt like the ground had been ripped out from under me, leaving me floating in a world filled with medical jargon, specialists, and unfamiliar terms. But as the days turned into weeks and the weeks turned into years, I learned that the strength I needed was always there, waiting to be discovered.

You, too, will find that strength. In the moments when you feel powerless, when the challenges seem insurmountable, you'll discover a well of resilience that carries you through. And it's not just about finding that strength for yourself—it's about using it to become an advocate for your child, to fight for the care they need, and to make sure they are seen and valued in a world that often overlooks them.

One of the most important lessons I've learned over the years is that we cannot do this alone. As much as we wish we could be everything for our children, there are times when we need to lean on others—whether it's medical professionals, therapists, support groups, or other parents walking similar paths. Advocacy became my lifeline, and it will be yours, too. Learning how to speak up for my child, how to navigate the complex medical and educational systems, and how to find the right resources was a crucial part of this journey.

But I didn't do it alone. I found community in support groups, both online and in person. Connecting with other parents who understood my situation gave me the strength to keep going, even when the road felt impossibly hard. The sense of not being alone, of knowing that there were others who understood the sleepless nights and the worry-filled days, gave me comfort and hope. Throughout this book, you'll find tips on how to build your own support network and ways to tap into the resources that are available to you.

**The Gift of Perspective**

Over the years, my perspective on life has changed dramatically. The early days of grief and fear have gradually given way to a deeper appreciation for the small moments of joy, the milestones that feel like miracles, and the unbreakable bond I share with my child. While I once mourned the life I thought we would have, I now cherish the life we do have. It's a life filled with challenges, yes, but also with extraordinary love and resilience. My hope for you is that you will come to find that same peace and perspective in your own journey.

I've written this book as both a guide and a companion. It's filled with practical advice—what I wish I had known 24 years ago—and stories from parents who have walked this path. But more than that, it's a testament to the power of love, the importance of hope, and the incredible strength we carry as caregivers. My goal is for this book to be a source of encouragement on the difficult days, a reminder that you are doing an incredible job, and that you and your child are deserving of all the love and support the world can offer.

### A Journey of Hope and Resilience

This is not just your journey—it's your child's journey, too. Together, you are navigating a path that will shape both of your lives in unexpected ways. And while the road ahead may be filled with challenges, it's also filled with hope. Hope that your child will receive the care they need. Hope that you will find strength in the most difficult moments. Hope that your family will thrive, even in the face of adversity.

As you turn the pages of this book, I want you to feel a sense of connection—to know that there is a community of parents and caregivers who understand what you are going through, and who are here to offer support. I have walked this road for over two decades, and though it hasn't always been easy, it has been filled with lessons of love, courage, and growth. You, too, will find your way, and I hope that the advice, stories, and insights in this book help guide you on your journey.

You are stronger than you realize, and the love you carry for your child is more powerful than you know. Together, we will face the challenges, celebrate the victories, and continue to find hope in even the smallest moments. Thank you for allowing me to share my journey with you. I hope that this book becomes a beacon of hope, a source of strength, and a reminder that no matter how difficult the road, you are not alone.

*-Shae Freeman*

About the Author:

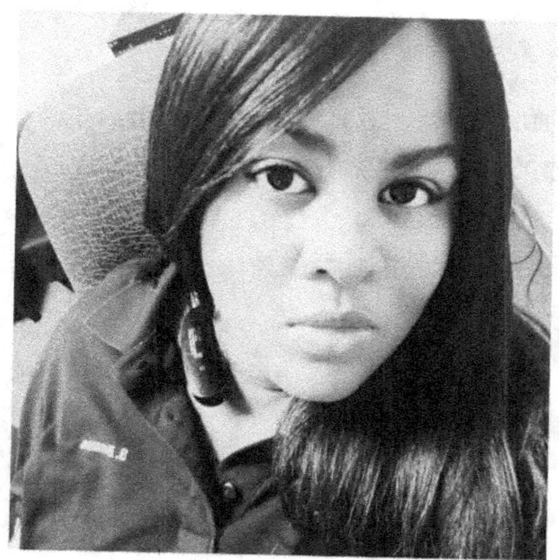

Shae Freeman is the proud owner and Training Director of Community Responders LLC. With a career spanning over two decades, she has dedicated her life to serving and educating others. As a paramedic with a local fire department in Arizona, Shae brings real-world experience to her work, ensuring every piece of advice and training she provides is practical and lifesaving.

Since 2004, Shae has also been a passionate freelance writer, crafting articles on a wide range of topics that have been published and appreciated by many. For the past 17 years, she has had the privilege of teaching CPR and other critical emergency courses, empowering countless individuals to respond confidently in emergencies.

Above all, Shae is a proud mother of three wonderful young men who inspire her daily. Her life's purpose is to make a positive impact, whether through her writing, her work as a paramedic, or her role as an instructor. She hopes her journey and insights will inspire readers and provide valuable knowledge to enhance their own lives.

## Disclaimer

Before we dive in, it's important to note that this ebook is not meant to replace your doctor's advice. Always follow your healthcare provider's recommendations and consult them for any medical concerns. Now, let's get started on this journey together!

# CHAPTER 1 THE DIAGNOSIS DAY—A TURNING POINT IN YOUR JOURNEY

The day you learn that your child has a rare condition is one that marks a profound shift in your life. It's a moment that leaves you feeling vulnerable, confused, and often overwhelmed. For many parents, this day feels like a blur—filled with medical jargon, tests, and discussions that are hard to process in the moment. You may be struggling with shock, grief, and fear, all while trying to grasp what the future will hold for your child. This chapter dives deep into the emotional and practical aspects of that pivotal moment, offering insights on how to cope, what steps to take next, and how to find support in the early days after diagnosis.

### The Emotional Rollercoaster: Navigating Shock and Grief

When you first hear the diagnosis, it's common to feel an overwhelming sense of disbelief. Many parents describe this moment as surreal, almost as if they are watching it happen to someone else. The shock is often accompanied by feelings of confusion—how could this happen? Why my child? This initial response is normal, and part of the emotional journey that unfolds as parents begin to process the reality of their child's condition.

Common Emotional Reactions

1. Denial: For many parents, the first reaction is denial. You may find yourself thinking, "This can't be true" or "There must be some mistake." Denial acts as a

psychological buffer, protecting you from the full weight of the situation until you are ready to confront it.

2. Anger and Guilt: As the diagnosis sinks in, it's common to feel a sense of anger or guilt. You might ask yourself, "Why my child?" or feel guilty, wondering if there was something you could have done differently to prevent the condition. These emotions are part of the normal grieving process, and it's important to allow yourself to feel them without judgment. Grief counselors explain that guilt is a natural response, especially for parents, as it reflects your deep desire to protect your child.

3. Bargaining and "What-If" Thinking: Many parents fall into a pattern of bargaining, mentally running through scenarios of what could have been done to change the outcome. You may start thinking about alternative paths, asking yourself questions like, "If we had caught this sooner, could things have been different?" This can be an exhausting mental loop, but it's another common reaction to loss—grieving for the future you had envisioned for your child.

4. Acceptance: Acceptance doesn't mean you are "okay" with the diagnosis, but rather that you come to terms with it. Acceptance is often a long process and can take months or even years. It's about reaching a point where you can begin to plan for the future, knowing that your child's condition is now part of their life—and yours.

**Coping with Overwhelm: Small Steps Forward**

The first few days after a diagnosis are often the hardest. Everything feels like it's happening too quickly, and yet time also seems to stand still. Parents often describe feeling like they are in a fog, unsure of what to do next.

What to Do First

1. Take Time to Process: It's crucial to give yourself permission to pause and process the news. While the medical team may be eager to move forward with treatments or interventions, don't feel pressured to rush into decisions before you are emotionally ready. Take a day or two to sit with the information and allow yourself to experience your emotions.

2. Ask for Clarification: Don't hesitate to ask your medical team for clarification on the diagnosis. Doctors often use complex terminology, and it's important that you fully understand what the diagnosis means for your child. Write down any questions you have, no matter how small or specific, and ask for simple explanations. Many hospitals have patient liaisons or genetic counselors who can help you understand the medical details in clearer terms.

3. Seek a Second Opinion: It's natural to want confirmation of the diagnosis from another specialist, especially if the condition is rare or difficult to treat. Seeking a second opinion can provide peace of mind and help you feel more confident in your child's care plan. Many leading children's hospitals, such as the Children's Hospital of Philadelphia (CHOP) or Mayo Clinic, specialize in rare conditions and can offer valuable insights.

4. Lean on Your Support System: This is not a time to go it alone. Reach out to trusted family members or friends who can offer emotional support. Even if they don't fully understand what you're going through, having someone there to listen can provide a sense of relief. You may also want to consider joining a support group for parents of children with rare conditions—many organizations, such as NORD and Genetic Alliance, offer both in-person and online communities.

## Understanding the Grieving Process for Parents

When a child is diagnosed with a rare condition, parents often experience a form of grief that is sometimes referred to as "ambiguous loss". Unlike the grief of losing a loved one, ambiguous loss refers to the mourning of an imagined future —a life you envisioned for your child that may now look very different. This type of grief is complex because, while your child is still with you, the dreams you held for them may feel unreachable.

Grief therapists explain that the grieving process for parents in these situations involves both acceptance of the diagnosis and adjusting to a new reality. It's important to give yourself permission to grieve for what you've lost, while also holding onto hope for what is still possible.

Stages of Grief Specific to Rare Conditions

1. Grieving the Life You Imagined: For many parents, one of the most challenging aspects of the diagnosis is letting go of the life you had envisioned for your child. This might include expectations of certain milestones, like graduating high school or getting married, which now seem uncertain. It's okay to mourn these imagined futures, but it's also important to remind yourself that your child can still live a fulfilling and meaningful life.

2. Living with Uncertainty: Rare conditions often come with a great deal of uncertainty. You may not have a clear prognosis or may be told that your child's condition is unpredictable. Learning to live with this uncertainty is one of the most difficult aspects of navigating a rare diagnosis. Many parents find comfort in focusing on the present—taking each day as it comes,

rather than trying to predict what the future will hold.

3. Hope for the Future: While the initial diagnosis may feel devastating, many parents find that over time, they begin to adjust to their new normal. Hope takes on new forms—hope for small victories, for moments of joy, and for the possibility of future medical advancements. Research into rare diseases is advancing every year, and staying informed about new treatments can provide a sense of hope that the future may bring unexpected possibilities.

**Practical First Steps: Navigating the Medical System**

Once the initial shock of the diagnosis begins to wear off, the next challenge is navigating the medical system. Rare conditions often require specialized care, and it's important to ensure that you are working with a medical team that has experience in treating your child's condition.

Key Steps to Take in the First Weeks After Diagnosis

1. Research Specialists: Look for doctors or clinics that specialize in your child's condition. Many rare diseases require multi-disciplinary care, involving specialists like geneticists, neurologists, and cardiologists. Hospitals such as Boston Children's Hospital and Cincinnati Children's Hospital are known for their expertise in treating complex pediatric conditions.

2. Join a Patient Advocacy Organization: Organizations like the National Organization for Rare Disorders (NORD) offer a wealth of resources, from medical information to patient advocacy tools. These organizations can help you connect with other families, find specialized care, and even access financial assistance for treatments.

3. Keep Detailed Records: One of the most important

things you can do in the early days after diagnosis is to start keeping detailed records of your child's medical history. This includes keeping copies of test results, medical reports, and any correspondence with doctors. Having an organized medical binder will help you stay on top of your child's care, especially when working with multiple specialists.

The diagnosis day is just the beginning of a long and sometimes difficult journey. While the road ahead may feel uncertain, it's important to remember that you don't have to walk it alone. As you process the news and begin to navigate the medical system, lean on the resources available to you—from support groups and advocacy organizations to your friends and family. In the chapters ahead, we'll explore more practical steps to take, from advocating for your child's care to finding financial support and long-term planning for their future.

Your emotions in these early days are valid, and it's okay to feel overwhelmed. But remember: resilience doesn't come from never feeling lost, but from finding your way forward, one step at a time.

# CHAPTER 2: IT'S OKAY TO FEEL WHAT YOU'RE FEELING—NAVIGATING COMPLEX EMOTIONS

The emotional aftermath of receiving a rare diagnosis for your child can feel overwhelming. You may find yourself cycling through an array of intense emotions—grief, guilt, anger, fear, and sometimes even relief in finally having an answer. It's important to recognize that these feelings are not only valid but also an essential part of the process. This chapter delves deeper into the complex emotional journey, offering guidance on how to manage your feelings, and introducing techniques for coping with the mental and emotional toll that comes with caring for a child with a rare condition.

## The Weight of Grief: Mourning the Life You Imagined

When a child is diagnosed with a rare condition, it often triggers a deep sense of grief. This grief is unique because it may not stem from the loss of a child, but rather from the loss of the life you imagined for them. This is sometimes referred to as "living grief"—grieving for the future that may never come.

Parents may mourn milestones they once envisioned for their child, such as running on the playground, going to prom, or achieving academic success. While these events might still happen, they may look different than you had expected. Understanding this grief and allowing yourself to feel it fully is essential to healing.

Strategies for Processing Grief:

1. Acknowledge the Loss: It's important to validate your feelings of grief. Just because your child is still with you does not mean that you haven't experienced a loss. Mourning the life you envisioned for your child does not diminish your love for them. Acknowledging your loss is the first step toward acceptance.

2. Connect with Others Who Understand: Grief shared is often easier to bear. Seek out parents or support groups who understand the unique grief that comes with raising a child with a rare condition. This shared experience can provide immense comfort and help reduce feelings of isolation. Organizations such as The Compassionate Friends and NORD offer both online and in-person support groups where parents can share their emotions.

3. Create New Dreams: It's okay to let go of the dreams you once held and begin imagining new ones. While the future may look different, your child's life is still full of potential. Finding new ways to celebrate their victories, no matter how small, can help shift your focus toward the possibilities that still lie ahead.

### Dealing with Guilt: Letting Go of 'What-Ifs'

Guilt is a pervasive emotion for many parents after receiving their child's diagnosis. You may wonder if you missed early signs of the condition or if you could have done something differently. This type of guilt often stems from a deep desire to protect your child from harm, and when that protection feels out of your control, guilt fills the void.

Managing Guilt:

1. Challenge Your Inner Critic: Guilt often arises from

unrealistic expectations we place on ourselves. You might find yourself thinking, "I should have seen this coming" or "I should have done more." These thoughts are rooted in the false belief that you could have changed the outcome. When you find yourself falling into this mindset, challenge these thoughts by reminding yourself that you did the best you could with the information you had at the time.

2. Focus on What You Can Control: Instead of dwelling on what you think you could have done in the past, focus on what you can do now. You are your child's greatest advocate, and your actions going forward—seeking the best care, advocating for their needs, and offering them unconditional love—are what truly matter.

3. Share Your Guilt: It's common to feel guilty about discussing your feelings of guilt, but sharing them can be incredibly healing. Whether it's with a therapist, a support group, or a trusted friend, talking about your guilt openly can reduce its power over you. You may find that many other parents share similar feelings, and realizing you're not alone in your guilt can be a source of comfort.

**Fear of the Unknown: Coping with Uncertainty**

Rare conditions often come with many unknowns. You may not have a clear prognosis, and you might be unsure of what your child's future will look like. Living with this uncertainty can create a constant undercurrent of anxiety and fear, as you may feel like you're always waiting for the next medical crisis or developmental setback.

Managing Fear and Anxiety:

1. Mindfulness Practices: One of the most effective ways

to manage the anxiety that comes with uncertainty is to practice mindfulness. Mindfulness encourages you to stay present in the current moment, rather than worrying about what may or may not happen in the future. Simple techniques such as focusing on your breath, grounding exercises, or guided meditations can help reduce feelings of overwhelm.

2. Focus on the Present: While it's natural to worry about the future, it's important to also live in the present. Celebrate today's achievements, no matter how small. Whether it's your child saying a new word, taking a step, or simply having a good day, focusing on the present helps shift your attention away from fear.

3. Prepare, Don't Predict: It's easy to fall into the trap of trying to predict every possible outcome for your child's condition. Instead, focus on being prepared. Have a plan in place for potential medical emergencies or developmental challenges, but don't dwell on them. Knowing you are prepared will give you peace of mind without becoming consumed by fear.

**Anger and Frustration: Finding Healthy Outlets**

Anger is another common emotional response to your child's diagnosis. You may feel angry at the world, at the healthcare system, or even at yourself. It's important to recognize that anger, like guilt, is a natural part of the emotional process. The key is finding healthy ways to express that anger so it doesn't consume you.

Healthy Ways to Process Anger:

1. Physical Activity: Physical movement is one of the best ways to release pent-up anger. Whether it's going for a run, practicing yoga, or even taking a walk, moving your

body helps to release the adrenaline that builds up with anger and frustration.

2. Creative Outlets: Many parents find that creative expression helps them process their emotions. Writing, painting, or even playing music can provide an outlet for your feelings of anger and frustration. These creative activities don't need to be shared with others—they're simply a way for you to release and process your emotions in a productive way.

3. Talking About It: Find someone you trust and talk through your anger. Whether it's a therapist, a friend, or another parent who has been through something similar, voicing your frustrations helps you process and release them.

### Acceptance: The Long Road to Peace

Acceptance doesn't mean you are "okay" with your child's condition, but it does mean coming to terms with the reality of the situation. Acceptance often comes slowly, and it's common to move in and out of acceptance over time. This doesn't mean you're failing—it's simply part of the process. Many parents describe the journey to acceptance as one of gradual healing, where moments of peace become more frequent over time.

How to Foster Acceptance:

1. Practice Self-Compassion: Acceptance often begins with self-compassion. Recognize that this journey is difficult and that you are doing the best you can. Be gentle with yourself when you have hard days, and allow yourself the space to heal at your own pace.

2. Embrace the New Normal: Over time, you will begin to adjust to your new normal. While this may not be the life you envisioned, it is still a life filled

with love, connection, and meaning. Finding ways to embrace your child's unique journey, and celebrating their achievements, can help foster a sense of peace and acceptance.

3. Stay Connected to Your Community: Acceptance is often made easier when you have a strong support system. Stay connected with other parents, your healthcare team, and support groups. These connections remind you that you are not alone, and that many others have walked this path before you.

### Seeking Professional Help: Therapists and Counselors Who Can Help

While it's normal to experience a wide range of emotions after your child's diagnosis, there are times when professional help is needed. If you find that your emotions are interfering with your ability to care for your child, maintain relationships, or manage daily life, it may be time to seek help from a mental health professional.

Many parents find that working with a therapist who specializes in grief, trauma, or chronic illness can provide invaluable support. A therapist can help you process your emotions, develop coping strategies, and provide you with tools to manage the stress and anxiety that often accompany caring for a child with a rare condition.

The emotions you experience after your child's diagnosis are complex and valid. Grief, guilt, anger, and fear are all natural responses to the life-altering news you've received. By allowing yourself to fully feel these emotions, and by finding healthy ways to process them, you can begin the journey toward healing and acceptance.

Remember, you are not alone in this journey. Many parents have walked this path before you, and there is a community of support waiting to help. As you navigate the emotional ups and downs, know that it's okay to feel what you're feeling. With time, support, and self-compassion, you will find your way forward.

# CHAPTER 3: BECOMING YOUR CHILD'S VOICE—ADVOCATING FOR THEIR NEEDS

When your child is diagnosed with a rare condition, you quickly realize that you are not only their caregiver but also their strongest advocate. Whether in medical settings, at school, or with insurance providers, your voice will often be the one guiding and pushing for the best possible care and opportunities for your child. Advocacy can feel daunting at first, but with time and practice, you will learn how to confidently navigate these systems and effectively communicate your child's needs. This chapter delves deeper into becoming an empowered advocate for your child, providing detailed strategies, resources, and real-life stories from parents who have successfully advocated for their children.

## The Importance of Advocacy: Why Your Voice Matters

Rare conditions often come with unique challenges that require individualized care. As a parent, you are the most consistent figure in your child's life, making you the best person to advocate for them. You understand their needs, behaviors, and responses better than anyone else, and you have the power to ensure they receive the appropriate care, education, and accommodations. Advocacy goes beyond medical settings—it can also mean advocating for educational resources, insurance coverage, social services, and emotional support.

Your Role as an Advocate

    1. Medical Advocate: You will often act as the liaison

between your child and medical professionals. This includes not only asking questions but also ensuring your child's needs and concerns are heard and understood by doctors, nurses, and specialists. In cases involving complex conditions, you may need to seek second opinions or push for more comprehensive treatment options.

2. Educational Advocate: Whether your child attends public or private school or is homeschooled, you will need to ensure they receive an education that accommodates their specific needs. This often involves collaborating with teachers, administrators, and special education professionals to develop an Individualized Education Plan (IEP) or 504 Plan (in the U.S.).

3. Financial Advocate: Navigating the financial side of your child's condition is a significant part of advocacy. You will need to communicate with insurance companies, apply for financial assistance programs, and find ways to cover treatments, therapies, and adaptive equipment that are essential for your child's well-being.

### Advocating in Medical Settings: Navigating the Healthcare System

Navigating the healthcare system can be incredibly complex, especially when dealing with a rare condition that few doctors may have encountered. Advocating for the best medical care means educating yourself about your child's condition, preparing for medical appointments, and ensuring that healthcare providers are on the same page regarding your child's treatment plan.

How to Prepare for Medical Appointments

1. Be Informed: Take time to educate yourself about your child's condition. Research trusted medical sources, join

patient advocacy groups, and stay informed about the latest developments in treatments or therapies. While doctors are experts in medicine, you are the expert on your child. The more informed you are, the better you can advocate for their needs.

2. Bring a List of Questions: Medical appointments can feel overwhelming, and it's easy to forget questions in the moment. Before each appointment, prepare a list of specific questions about your child's treatment, prognosis, medications, and therapies. Asking for clarification or second opinions is perfectly normal and necessary to ensure your child is receiving the best care.

3. Keep Detailed Records: Maintaining a comprehensive medical binder or digital record for your child's care is crucial. This should include diagnoses, test results, treatment plans, medication lists, and any correspondence with doctors. Being organized helps you stay on top of your child's care, especially if you're dealing with multiple specialists or complex treatment plans.

### The Power of Second Opinions

Don't hesitate to seek a second opinion, especially if you feel unsure about a diagnosis or treatment plan. For rare conditions, many specialists may be involved, and it's common for parents to consult multiple experts to ensure they are considering all available options. Second opinions can confirm a diagnosis, offer alternative treatment paths, or introduce new perspectives that your current medical team may not have considered.

Several renowned hospitals, such as the Mayo Clinic, Cleveland Clinic, and Boston Children's Hospital, have programs specifically designed for complex cases and rare diseases. These institutions may offer more specialized care or cutting-edge treatments that are not available at smaller or regional hospitals.

## Educational Advocacy: Ensuring Your Child's Needs Are Met

Advocating for your child's education can be one of the most important aspects of ensuring they reach their full potential. Whether your child has cognitive, physical, or developmental challenges, their educational environment needs to adapt to their unique learning style and needs. In the U.S., legal protections like the Individuals with Disabilities Education Act (IDEA) and Section 504 of the Rehabilitation Act provide children with disabilities the right to a free and appropriate public education, including any necessary accommodations.

## Developing an Individualized Education Plan (IEP)

An IEP is a legally binding document that outlines specific accommodations, goals, and services your child will receive in the school setting. Working with a team of educators, school administrators, and therapists, you will help create this plan to ensure your child's needs are met in the classroom. Here's how to approach IEP meetings:

1. Know Your Rights: Under IDEA, you have the right to participate in your child's IEP development. Schools are required to provide appropriate accommodations, therapies, and services that meet your child's unique needs. Familiarize yourself with IDEA provisions to ensure the school complies with the law.

2. Collaborate with Educators: IEP meetings are collaborative efforts between you, the school, and other professionals. Be prepared to advocate for services you believe are essential for your child's success, whether that's speech therapy, occupational therapy, or a classroom aide.

3. Set Measurable Goals: IEPs should include specific, measurable goals for your child's academic and personal

development. These goals should be updated regularly, and you have the right to request revisions or additional services if your child is not meeting their goals.

## 504 Plans: Accommodating Children with Disabilities

For children who may not qualify for an IEP but still require accommodations, a 504 Plan ensures they receive the support they need. A 504 Plan focuses more on providing equal access rather than specialized instruction. This could include classroom accommodations like extended time on tests, assistive technology, or modified seating arrangements.

## Financial Advocacy: Navigating Insurance and Assistance Programs

Healthcare costs for children with rare conditions can be overwhelming. Many treatments, therapies, and adaptive devices are expensive, and insurance coverage is not always guaranteed. As a financial advocate, your role is to navigate the complex world of insurance policies, financial assistance programs, and grants to ensure your child's medical expenses are covered.

Understanding Health Insurance

Health insurance policies can be difficult to navigate, especially when dealing with rare and complex conditions. Here are key steps to take:

1. Know What's Covered: Take time to thoroughly read and understand your health insurance policy. Pay attention to what treatments, medications, and therapies are covered. Some insurance companies may deny coverage for certain treatments, labeling them "experimental" or "non-essential," even if they are vital for your child.

2. File Appeals: If your insurance provider denies coverage

for a treatment or therapy, don't give up. Many denials can be overturned through the appeals process. Work with your child's medical team to gather documentation that supports the necessity of the treatment, and file an appeal with your insurance company.

3. Look for Supplemental Programs: In addition to your primary insurance, look for supplemental insurance programs or government programs like Medicaid or Children's Health Insurance Program (CHIP). These programs may cover services that your primary insurance doesn't, especially if your child qualifies for disability-based benefits.

## Seeking Financial Assistance

Beyond insurance, many nonprofit organizations provide financial aid to families caring for children with rare conditions. These organizations can help with the costs of medical treatments, travel for specialized care, and adaptive equipment. Some resources include:

- UnitedHealthcare Children's Foundation: Provides grants to help cover medical costs not covered by insurance.

- Miracle Flights: Offers free flights to families who need to travel long distances for medical care.

- NORD Patient Assistance Programs: Offers financial aid to families dealing with rare diseases, including help with medications and diagnostic testing.

## How to Build Confidence as an Advocate

Advocating for your child can feel intimidating at first, especially when you're dealing with medical professionals, educators, or insurance representatives who may have more experience or expertise in their fields. However, it's important to remember that you are the expert when it comes to your child's needs. With time, practice, and the right resources, you will become more confident in your advocacy efforts.

## Empower Yourself with Knowledge

The more informed you are about your child's condition, the more confidently you can advocate for them. Join rare disease support groups, attend conferences or webinars, and read up on the latest research in your child's specific condition. Many advocacy organizations provide free educational resources for parents, helping them navigate the complexities of rare diseases.

## Find Your Support System

Being an advocate can feel overwhelming at times, and it's essential to have a support system in place. Whether it's a local parent group, an online community, or professional support from patient advocacy organizations, having others who understand your journey can provide both emotional support and practical advice.

Becoming your child's advocate is a role you may not have expected, but it's one of the most important things you will do for them. Your voice matters

# CHAPTER 4: NAVIGATING THE MEDICAL MAZE—FINDING THE RIGHT CARE AND RESOURCES

Navigating the medical system for a child with a rare condition can feel overwhelming. The healthcare system is often complex and can be particularly challenging when dealing with a rare disease that few doctors may be familiar with. This chapter will provide a detailed roadmap for parents on how to effectively manage their child's healthcare, from finding the right specialists to advocating for proper care, to staying organized with medical information.

## Understanding Rare Diseases and the Healthcare System

A rare disease is defined as a condition that affects fewer than 200,000 people in the United States. While this might not sound like a large number, there are over 7,000 rare diseases identified, collectively impacting around 30 million Americans. Many rare diseases are genetic, chronic, and progressive, and for the majority, there are no cures—only treatments to manage symptoms. Because of their rarity, even healthcare providers may have limited experience with certain conditions.

## The Role of Specialists

For many rare conditions, the treatment often requires input from various medical specialists. These can include:

- Geneticists: Specialize in conditions related to genetic mutations or anomalies.

- Neurologists: Treat conditions affecting the brain and

nervous system.

- Endocrinologists: Manage hormonal and metabolic disorders, common in many rare diseases.
- Cardiologists or Pulmonologists: Monitor heart or lung-related issues that may arise as a result of certain rare conditions.

Many rare diseases require multidisciplinary care, which means you may need to work with a team of doctors who collaborate across different areas of expertise. Some of the best hospitals for treating rare conditions have established centers that offer multidisciplinary approaches, such as the National Institutes of Health (NIH) Clinical Center or Mayo Clinic, where teams of specialists work together to manage complex diseases.

### Finding the Right Doctors and Hospitals

Choosing the right healthcare team is one of the most important decisions you'll make for your child. Here are several ways to ensure your child is receiving the best care:

1. Research Specialized Hospitals: Many hospitals specialize in specific rare conditions or offer comprehensive care centers for managing them. For example, the Children's Hospital of Philadelphia (CHOP) and Boston Children's Hospital are renowned for their expertise in pediatric rare diseases, while Cleveland Clinic and Johns Hopkins Hospital are well-known for their work with adults with rare diseases.

2. Get Recommendations from Advocacy Groups: Patient advocacy groups like Global Genes and NORD often maintain databases of healthcare professionals who specialize in particular rare diseases. These groups can connect you with experts, direct you to clinical trials, or provide up-to-date treatment options.

3. Telemedicine and Rare Disease Clinics: In the age of digital healthcare, telemedicine has become an invaluable resource for families who live far from major hospitals. Many hospitals now offer virtual consultations, allowing you to connect with specialists who might not be located nearby. Several major hospitals also have dedicated rare disease clinics, providing targeted expertise.

### Preparing for Medical Appointments: Maximizing Your Time with Doctors

Because rare disease appointments can involve multiple specialists, extensive testing, and difficult-to-understand medical terminology, it's essential to make the most out of each appointment.

Tips for Preparing for Appointments

1. Bring a Comprehensive Medical History: Ensure that you have all relevant documentation, including your child's diagnosis, test results, and previous treatments. A well-organized medical binder can help you keep track of your child's condition and ensure that all specialists are informed.

2. Develop a List of Questions: Each appointment will likely bring new information, and it can be overwhelming to keep track of it all. Preparing a list of questions beforehand can help you focus on key issues such as:

    - What is the current status of my child's condition?

    - Are there any new treatments or therapies we should consider?

    - How do we proceed with care if symptoms

worsen?

Don't hesitate to ask for clarification on anything you don't understand.

3. Record the Appointment: If your doctor allows it, consider recording the conversation or taking detailed notes. This can help you revisit important information later and ensure that you didn't miss any critical details. Many parents find that having a trusted friend or family member attend appointments with them can also help them process information more effectively.

**Managing and Organizing Medical Information**

One of the most difficult aspects of managing a rare disease is keeping track of medical records, test results, doctor's notes, and treatment plans. Being organized can save time, reduce stress, and ensure your child's care is consistent, even when multiple specialists are involved.

Create a Medical Binder or Digital File

A medical binder or secure digital file is a great way to keep all important documents in one place. Key items to include:

- A summary of your child's medical history
- Test results (bloodwork, imaging, etc.)
- Medication lists, including dosages and side effects
- Contact information for all doctors and specialists
- Notes from appointments
- Copies of insurance claims, approvals, or denials

There are also several apps and digital platforms available that allow you to store and manage medical records online. Many hospitals offer patient portals that give you direct access to your child's test results, prescriptions, and doctor's notes. Services like MyChart or CareZone can help consolidate all of your child's medical information into one secure place.

## The Importance of Early Intervention

For children with rare conditions, early intervention can make a significant difference in their overall development. Early intervention refers to services and support systems that can help children with disabilities or developmental delays. These services can include physical therapy, occupational therapy, speech therapy, and educational support.

Accessing Early Intervention Services

1. Birth to Age 3: In the U.S., early intervention services are often available for children from birth to age 3 through state-funded programs. Contact your state's Early Intervention Program (EIP) to begin the evaluation process. If your child qualifies, they will receive services tailored to their needs, such as therapy sessions or family support services.

2. Ages 3 to 5: After age 3, services are typically provided through the public school system under IDEA Part B. Even if your child is not yet in school, the local school district may offer services to help them prepare for kindergarten or primary school.

3. Ages 5 and Up: Once your child enters school, they may qualify for additional services through an Individualized Education Plan (IEP) or 504 Plan to accommodate their learning and developmental needs.

The earlier these services are implemented, the better the chance for long-term developmental improvements. Early intervention has been shown to improve outcomes in children with a range of developmental disabilities, providing them with the tools and skills necessary to thrive.

## Clinical Trials and Research: Exploring Cutting-Edge Treatments

For some rare diseases, standard treatment options are limited, which is why many parents consider clinical trials as a potential option for their child's care. Clinical trials can provide access to experimental treatments and cutting-edge therapies that aren't yet widely available.

How to Find Clinical Trials

- ClinicalTrials.gov: This government-run website provides a database of clinical trials being conducted around the world. It allows you to search for trials based on your child's condition, location, and the type of treatment being tested.

- Patient Advocacy Groups: Many rare disease advocacy organizations, such as NORD, regularly post information about ongoing clinical trials and studies. These organizations often work closely with research institutions and pharmaceutical companies, providing families with access to the latest developments.

- Hospital Referrals: Your child's medical team can also guide you to appropriate clinical trials. Major hospitals like the National Institutes of Health (NIH) run their own research trials and may offer early access to new therapies.

### Pros and Cons of Clinical Trials

Clinical trials can provide access to new treatments, but they also come with risks. It's important to weigh the potential benefits and challenges of enrolling your child in a trial:

- Benefits: Clinical trials can offer access to innovative treatments that may not be available elsewhere. Your child's participation could also contribute to broader scientific research that helps others in the future.

- Risks: Because clinical trials involve experimental treatments, there may be risks involved, including unknown side effects. It's important to fully understand the trial's goals, potential risks, and how they align with your child's needs before making a decision.

### Caring for Yourself as a Medical Advocate

It's easy to focus entirely on your child's needs and neglect your own well-being. However, caring for a child with a rare disease can be physically and emotionally draining. Taking care of your own health—both mental and physical—ensures that you can continue advocating for your child effectively.

Preventing Caregiver Burnout

1. Accept Help: Don't be afraid to lean on your support system—family, friends, or even professional caregivers —when you need a break. No one can handle everything alone.

2. Therapy for Caregivers: Speaking to a counselor or joining a support group specifically for caregivers can be a vital outlet for processing the stress and emotional burden that comes with caregiving.

3. Mindfulness and Stress Relief: Incorporate small moments of self-care into your routine, such as mindfulness exercises, meditation, or journaling. Taking even a few minutes a day for yourself can help reduce feelings of overwhelm.

Navigating the medical maze is no easy feat, but it's an essential part of advocating for your child. By learning to communicate with doctors, staying organized, researching advanced treatment options, and tapping into support systems, you can provide the best care possible for your child with a rare condition. Remember, you are your child's greatest champion, and the steps you take will ensure they receive the care they deserve.

# CHAPTER 5: THE POWER OF COMMUNITY SUPPORT —BUILDING A NETWORK OF HELP AND HOPE

When caring for a child with a rare condition, feelings of isolation can be overwhelming. Families may feel as though they are facing unique struggles that others cannot fully understand. However, the truth is that a vibrant, supportive community exists—both online and in-person—dedicated to helping parents of children with rare diseases. Finding and connecting with this community can offer emotional support, practical advice, and essential resources. In this chapter, we'll explore the power of community support, how to access these networks, and the practical benefits they provide for families facing the challenges of rare diseases.

## Why Community Support is Crucial

Caring for a child with a rare disease can bring about a wide range of challenges—medical, financial, emotional, and logistical. Often, these hurdles are ones that are difficult to explain to those who aren't directly familiar with rare diseases. Support from others who are walking the same path can be immensely valuable, and in many cases, it is other parents and caregivers who provide the most impactful help.

Emotional Benefits of Community Support

1. **Shared Experiences**: Being part of a community of parents and caregivers who understand your challenges can provide immense emotional relief. By sharing your story, you realize that you are not alone. Other

families can offer validation for the unique emotional experiences that arise from managing a rare condition.

2. **Reducing Isolation**: Rare diseases, by nature, affect small populations, which can make parents feel as if they are living in an isolated world. Online and in-person support groups help reduce this isolation by connecting families from across the globe who are facing similar struggles. Parents can share their experiences, offer advice, and even celebrate small victories together.

3. **Resilience and Hope**: Seeing other families cope with and manage rare diseases can inspire resilience and hope. Witnessing stories of survival, advocacy, and success can provide strength during difficult moments, and can offer a roadmap for navigating the path ahead.

Practical Benefits of Community Support

1. **Access to Information**: Many rare diseases have limited research, but online communities often share the most current information available about treatments, clinical trials, and specialists. Parents may find valuable insights about medication side effects, home care strategies, and therapies that have worked for others.

2. **Problem Solving**: Parents and caregivers are often creative problem-solvers. When you connect with others in a similar situation, you may learn new strategies for managing symptoms, dealing with insurance companies, or advocating for better educational accommodations.

3. **Financial Assistance**: Many community organizations offer financial resources, such as grants, travel assistance, or help with medical equipment. Families often share information about programs that can help

offset the high costs associated with rare disease care.

## Finding Support Groups: Local and Online Communities

There are numerous ways to find a support group tailored to your specific needs. Whether you prefer in-person meetings or online forums, there are resources available to connect you with a broader community of families dealing with similar conditions.

## Local Support Groups

Local support groups offer the chance to build in-person relationships with others who understand your challenges. Meeting face-to-face can foster deeper connections and provide immediate emotional support. These groups often meet at hospitals, community centers, or schools and may include:

- **Condition-Specific Groups**: Many hospitals and clinics host support groups for specific rare conditions. If your child receives care at a large hospital or a specialized center, ask about local groups that meet to discuss similar medical issues.

- **Parent and Caregiver Groups**: Even if there are no condition-specific groups nearby, many communities offer general support groups for parents of children with disabilities or chronic illnesses. These groups may focus on coping strategies, self-care, or navigating the medical system.

## Online Support Groups and Platforms

The internet has dramatically expanded the ability of families to connect across long distances. Online support groups allow families to access help no matter where they live, and these communities are often filled with parents sharing their experiences, challenges, and solutions. Here are some of the most popular and trusted online support platforms:

1. **Facebook Groups**: There are thousands of Facebook groups specifically for families of children with rare diseases. These groups are often condition-specific and provide a forum where parents can ask questions, share experiences, and offer support to one another. Examples include groups like "Rare Disease Parents" or groups specifically dedicated to conditions such as cystic fibrosis or spinal muscular atrophy (SMA).

2. **RareConnect**: A platform hosted by EURORDIS (European Rare Disease Organization), RareConnect provides forums where individuals and families affected by rare diseases can connect. It offers multilingual support and allows for discussions on medical treatment, clinical trials, and emotional well-being.

3. **The Mighty**: This online community offers support for people dealing with health challenges, including rare diseases. The platform includes condition-specific forums where users can share stories, ask questions, and provide mutual support.

4. **Global Genes**: As one of the largest rare disease patient advocacy organizations, Global Genes hosts a wide range of online forums, webinars, and virtual events. It also connects families with local and regional resources.

5. **NORD Rare Disease Support**: The National Organization for Rare Disorders (NORD) offers access to patient and caregiver forums as well as information on advocacy, research, and financial support programs. NORD also hosts a "Rare Action Network," which connects families to local resources and events

### The Role of Nonprofit Organizations and Foundations

Nonprofit organizations play a vital role in supporting families affected by rare diseases. These organizations provide a wide range of services, including financial assistance, advocacy, education, and awareness. Many of these groups were founded by parents of children with rare diseases, and they understand the unique challenges that come with raising a child with a rare condition.

Types of Services Provided by Nonprofits

1. **Financial Assistance**: Many organizations provide grants to help cover the costs of medical treatments, therapies, travel for medical care, and even daily living expenses. For example, the **UnitedHealthcare Children's Foundation** offers financial grants to families facing medical hardships, while **Miracle Flights** provides free air travel for medical appointments.

2. **Education and Advocacy**: Nonprofit organizations often work to raise awareness about specific conditions and the broader rare disease community. They also provide educational materials for families and healthcare professionals, helping to bridge the gap between families and the medical community. **Global Genes** and **NORD** are two leading organizations in rare disease advocacy, offering resources for patient education and legislative advocacy.

3. **Research Funding**: Many nonprofit foundations focus on funding research for treatments and cures. The **Cystic Fibrosis Foundation**, for example, has been a leader in driving research for new treatments for cystic fibrosis. These organizations often collaborate with medical institutions and pharmaceutical companies to promote clinical trials and drug development.

Examples of Leading Nonprofit Organizations

1. **NORD (National Organization for Rare Disorders)**: NORD is a leading advocate for individuals with rare diseases. The organization provides information, support, and financial assistance, and advocates for research and policy changes on behalf of the rare disease community. NORD also offers patient assistance programs that help cover medical and prescription costs

2. **Global Genes**: Another key player in the rare disease space, Global Genes provides resources and educational tools for families, advocates for policy changes, and hosts a large annual summit for the rare disease community.

3. **The Assistance Fund (TAF)**: TAF helps families manage the high costs of treatment for chronic or life-threatening conditions by offering financial assistance to cover out-of-pocket costs for prescriptions, medical supplies, and insurance premiums.

### Grants, Travel Assistance, and Financial Aid

One of the most challenging aspects of managing a rare condition is the financial burden. Between medical bills, travel expenses, and specialized equipment, the costs can quickly become overwhelming. Fortunately, many organizations offer financial support specifically for families of children with rare diseases.

Travel Assistance Programs

For families who need to travel long distances to see specialists or participate in clinical trials, travel assistance programs can be a lifesaver. Some notable programs include:

- **Miracle Flights**: Provides free flights for families traveling to access medical care not available in their local area.

- **Angel Flight**: A volunteer-based program where private pilots provide free flights to families in need of medical transportation.

Grants for Medical Expenses

Many organizations provide financial grants to help cover the cost of medical treatments, therapies, and equipment. Some notable examples include:

- **UnitedHealthcare Children's Foundation (UHCCF)**: Offers financial grants to families to help pay for medical treatments and therapies not covered by insurance.

- **Ronald McDonald House Charities**: Offers free or low-cost housing to families traveling for medical care, helping ease the financial burden of travel and accommodations.

Connecting with a community of support can make a tremendous difference in the emotional and practical aspects of raising a child with a rare disease. Whether you seek in-person connections through local groups or prefer to engage with others online, these networks can provide essential resources, encouragement, and a sense of solidarity. With the right support in place, families can find strength, hope, and valuable tools to manage the challenges of living with a rare condition.

# CHAPTER 6: INSURANCE, FINANCIAL PLANNING, AND RESOURCES—SECURING YOUR CHILD'S FUTURE

Raising a child with a rare condition can be emotionally and financially taxing. The high cost of medical treatments, specialized therapies, equipment, and other necessities can quickly add up. In this chapter, we'll explore how to navigate health insurance, plan for long-term financial stability, and find additional resources to ensure your child receives the care they need. From understanding the intricacies of health insurance to applying for financial assistance programs, this chapter will provide you with the tools and knowledge necessary to secure a stable financial future for your child and family.

## The Financial Burden of Rare Diseases

Children with rare diseases often require specialized medical care, ongoing therapies, and expensive medications. According to research conducted by the **National Organization for Rare Disorders (NORD)**, the average family caring for a child with a rare disease spends significantly more on healthcare than the average family. These expenses often include frequent hospital visits, medical supplies, travel to see specialists, and sometimes experimental treatments not covered by insurance. The costs can quickly become overwhelming, making financial planning a crucial part of long-term care.

## Understanding Health Insurance and Rare Conditions

Health insurance plays a critical role in covering medical expenses for rare conditions, but understanding and navigating insurance policies can be challenging. Insurance providers may not cover specific treatments, therapies, or medications, particularly if they are deemed experimental or not part of a standard treatment plan for more common conditions. This section will help you understand how to make the most of your insurance coverage, appeal denials, and find supplementary programs that can fill in the gaps.

Navigating Your Health Insurance Plan

1. **Understand Your Coverage**: Review your health insurance plan thoroughly to understand what is and isn't covered. Look specifically at sections covering **specialist visits, hospitalizations, long-term care**, and **durable medical equipment** (such as wheelchairs or communication devices).

   - Some plans may have caps on physical therapy, occupational therapy, or speech therapy visits. If these therapies are critical for your child's development, it's important to understand the limits and how you can work around them.

   - Many rare conditions require medications that are expensive or newly developed, and these treatments may be listed as "experimental" by insurance companies. Be sure to check whether your child's medications are covered under your plan's **formulary**, and what the out-of-pocket costs will be if they aren't covered.

2. **Network vs. Out-of-Network Providers**: Many insurance plans have "in-network" providers—doctors and specialists who have agreed to work with the insurance company for reduced fees. If your child's care involves specialists that are out of network, your out-of-

pocket costs can increase significantly. Understanding these distinctions can help you determine whether you should pursue care in-network or seek **out-of-network benefits**.

3. **Health Savings Accounts (HSAs) and Flexible Spending Accounts (FSAs)**: If your insurance plan includes an **HSA** or **FSA**, take full advantage of it. These accounts allow you to set aside pre-tax money to pay for medical expenses, which can be used for co-pays, deductibles, medications, and certain therapies. Maximizing your contributions to these accounts each year can help offset the financial burden of ongoing care.

4. **Maximizing Benefits**: Some insurance policies offer case management services or a care coordinator who can help you navigate the complexities of coverage, find providers, and make the most of your benefits. These services are especially helpful when dealing with rare diseases that require complex, ongoing care.

## Filing Insurance Appeals

It's common for insurance companies to deny coverage for certain treatments or therapies, especially for rare conditions where treatment plans are not as standardized as they are for more common illnesses. However, a denied claim does not necessarily mean the end of the road.

Steps to Take When Filing an Appeal

1. **Request a Detailed Explanation**: When a claim is denied, the insurance company is required to provide a reason for the denial. Make sure you obtain this information in writing, as it will help guide your appeal.

2. **Gather Supporting Documentation**: Work with your child's medical team to gather documentation

supporting the need for the denied treatment or service. This may include letters from your child's doctors, medical records, and research articles showing the effectiveness of the treatment for your child's condition.

3. **Submit a Formal Appeal**: Insurance companies typically allow you to submit a formal appeal within a certain timeframe. The appeal should include a detailed explanation of why the treatment is necessary, along with the supporting documentation you've collected.

4. **Consider an External Review**: If your appeal is denied, you have the right to request an external review by an independent third party. This reviewer will examine the case and decide whether the insurance company should cover the treatment.

Appealing a denial can be a lengthy and frustrating process, but many families are successful in overturning initial denials, particularly when armed with documentation from their child's medical team. Advocacy organizations like **NORD** and **Global Genes** offer resources to help families navigate insurance denials and appeals.

## Medicaid and Supplemental Insurance

In addition to private health insurance, families of children with rare diseases may be eligible for **Medicaid** or other supplemental insurance programs, depending on income, disability status, and state regulations.

Medicaid and CHIP

- **Medicaid**: Medicaid is a federal and state-funded program that provides health coverage to low-income individuals, including children with disabilities. Unlike private insurance, Medicaid often provides more comprehensive coverage for long-term care, home health services, and therapies such as speech or occupational therapy. Many families turn to Medicaid for secondary insurance coverage to fill in the gaps left by private insurance.

- **Children's Health Insurance Program (CHIP)**: CHIP provides health insurance for children in families with income levels too high for Medicaid but too low to afford private insurance. CHIP covers doctor's visits, prescriptions, hospitalizations, and preventive care, which can help ease the financial burden on families.

## Medicare for Children with Disabilities

While **Medicare** is typically associated with the elderly, some children with disabilities are eligible for **Medicare** benefits, particularly if they are receiving **Social Security Disability Insurance (SSDI)** or **Supplemental Security Income (SSI)** benefits. If your child qualifies, Medicare can provide additional coverage for hospital care, doctor's visits, and certain therapies.

## Special Needs Trusts and Long-Term Financial Planning

Financial planning for a child with a rare disease requires not only managing current medical costs but also planning for the future. **Special Needs Trusts**, **ABLE accounts**, and other financial tools can help you protect your child's financial future while ensuring that they continue to receive the care and support they need throughout their lives.

## Special Needs Trusts (SNTs)

A **Special Needs Trust** is a legal arrangement that allows you to set aside money for your child's future care without jeopardizing their eligibility for government benefits like Medicaid or SSI. Funds in a special needs trust can be used to pay for a variety of services and needs, including:

- Medical care not covered by insurance
- Therapies, equipment, and assistive technologies
- Caregivers and in-home care
- Housing, transportation, and recreational activities

**Third-Party SNTs** are often set up by parents or relatives and are funded by gifts, inheritances, or life insurance policies. These funds can only be used for the benefit of the child with a disability, ensuring that they are cared for in the long term.

## ABLE Accounts

An **Achieving a Better Life Experience (ABLE) account** is a savings account designed for individuals with disabilities. Similar to a 529 college savings plan, ABLE accounts allow you to save money for disability-related expenses without affecting eligibility for government benefits. ABLE accounts can be used for a wide range of expenses, including:

- Housing and transportation
- Medical care and therapies
- Assistive technology
- Education and job training

The main benefit of an ABLE account is that the funds grow tax-free, and contributions up to a certain limit (depending on your state) do not affect eligibility for programs like SSI or Medicaid.

## Financial Assistance Programs and Grants

Beyond insurance and personal savings, many nonprofit organizations and government programs provide financial assistance to families dealing with rare conditions. These programs can help cover medical bills, travel costs, and even daily living expenses related to caring for a child with a rare disease.

Organizations Providing Financial Aid

1. **The Assistance Fund**: Provides financial assistance for out-of-pocket medical expenses, including medications and treatments that are not fully covered by insurance.

2. **UnitedHealthcare Children's Foundation (UHCCF)**: Offers medical grants to help families cover healthcare costs not covered by insurance. These grants can be used for surgeries, therapies, medications, and equipment.

3. **Miracle Flights**: Offers free flights to families who need to travel long distances for specialized medical care.

4. **NORD's RareCare® Assistance Programs**: NORD provides financial assistance for diagnostic testing, medications, and travel for medical appointments for individuals with rare diseases.

## State and Federal Programs

In addition to nonprofit organizations, state and federal programs offer support for families with children who have special healthcare needs:

- **Supplemental Security Income (SSI)**: SSI provides monthly financial benefits to families of children with disabilities. SSI eligibility is based on both the child's disability and family income level. The monthly benefits can help cover the costs of daily care, housing, and other essentials.

## Creating a Comprehensive Financial Plan for Your Child's Future

As a parent or caregiver to a child with a rare condition, planning for your child's future financial security is one of the most critical—and sometimes overwhelming—steps you can take. This process is multifaceted, combining elements such as maximizing insurance benefits, seeking financial assistance, planning for long-term care, and creating a structured estate plan. Securing your child's financial future may seem daunting, but careful preparation ensures that they will be well-supported throughout their life, even in your absence.

## Combining Health and Life Insurance

When structuring a financial plan for your child, it's crucial to integrate both health insurance and life insurance into your overall strategy. Health insurance will help manage the ongoing costs of medical care and treatments, while life insurance provides a financial safety net that can cover your child's expenses in the event of your death or incapacitation.

## Maximizing Health Insurance Benefits

Health insurance serves as the primary mechanism for paying for your child's healthcare needs, including doctor's visits, medications, surgeries, therapies, and medical equipment. Families should explore all options to maximize the benefits from their health insurance policies and ensure that they are taking full advantage of any available government assistance programs like **Medicaid**, **CHIP**, or **waiver programs** that can provide additional coverage beyond private insurance. Here's how to ensure you're optimizing health insurance benefits:

1. **Annual Plan Review**: Each year, review your insurance policy during the open enrollment period to ensure you are on the best plan for your child's specific needs. Make sure to consider changes in coverage, premium costs, and changes in the list of in-network providers.

2. **Prescription Coverage**: Given that many rare diseases require expensive medications, ensure that your plan has comprehensive prescription drug coverage. If your child's medications are not covered, inquire about applying for **compassionate use programs** or assistance

from pharmaceutical companies, which may provide drugs at discounted rates or even for free.

3. **Out-of-Pocket Costs**: Pay attention to deductibles, co-pays, and out-of-pocket maximums. Families often find it beneficial to keep a **health savings account (HSA)** or a **flexible spending account (FSA)** to manage these expenses. These accounts allow you to set aside pre-tax income to pay for medical expenses not covered by insurance, which can provide significant tax savings over time.

4. **Employer-Sponsored Health Insurance**: If your family has access to employer-sponsored health insurance, explore all available options, including **group insurance plans** that may offer more comprehensive coverage or have fewer restrictions compared to private individual plans. Some large companies even provide access to specialized programs for children with chronic illnesses.

### Supplementing with Life Insurance

While health insurance addresses your child's immediate medical needs, **life insurance** serves as a long-term financial safeguard. It ensures that, in the event of your death, there are funds available to support your child's care and living expenses. Two types of life insurance commonly used by families of children with special needs are:

1. **Term Life Insurance**: This type of policy provides coverage for a specified period (typically 10-30 years). It's generally more affordable than whole life insurance and is suitable for parents who want to ensure their child's needs are covered during their dependent years. The death benefit from a term life policy can be allocated to a special needs trust to cover ongoing medical or caregiving expenses.

2. **Whole Life Insurance**: Unlike term insurance, whole life insurance provides lifetime coverage and builds cash value over time. This can be an effective tool for families who want to ensure long-term financial support for their child well into adulthood. The cash value aspect of whole life insurance can also be accessed before death to pay for medical or caregiving costs if needed.

### Adding Riders for Long-Term Disability

Some insurance policies allow you to add **disability riders**, which provide additional benefits if your child becomes permanently disabled due to their condition. These riders can help cover long-term care costs, including residential facilities, specialized nursing care, or additional therapies that may not be fully covered by health insurance.

### Establishing Legal Guardianship

In many cases, children with rare diseases may require lifelong caregiving, even after they reach adulthood. Establishing legal guardianship is essential to ensure that your child's rights and needs are protected after they turn 18. Guardianship allows you (or a trusted individual) to make legal, financial, and healthcare decisions on behalf of your adult child. Here's how to approach this process:

1. **Petitioning for Guardianship**: Guardianship is granted by a court, and the process usually involves submitting medical records and a formal petition demonstrating that your child is unable to make decisions independently. Courts may also appoint a legal guardian ad litem to represent your child's interests during the process.

2. **Choosing a Successor Guardian**: If you are appointed as the legal guardian, it's crucial to name a successor

who will assume the role in the event of your death or incapacitation. This ensures that your child's care will continue without interruption.

3. **Alternatives to Full Guardianship**: Depending on your child's needs, limited guardianship may be more appropriate. This arrangement allows your child to maintain some independence while receiving support for specific decisions, such as financial or healthcare matters. Another option is a **power of attorney** or **conservatorship**, which grants specific decision-making authority without full guardianship.

# CHAPTER 7: PREPARING FOR THE FUTURE—PLANNING FOR YOUR CHILD'S LIFE AFTER YOU

One of the most challenging realities for parents of children with rare conditions is planning for the time when they can no longer provide direct care. The thought of what will happen to your child after you are no longer able to care for them can bring anxiety and uncertainty. However, with proper planning and the right resources, you can create a safety net that will ensure your child's needs continue to be met throughout their life. This chapter delves into strategies for future planning, from selecting a long-term caregiver to developing financial and legal plans that will protect your child in the years to come.

## The Emotional Aspect of Planning for the Future

Thinking about your child's future, particularly in a world where you are not present to care for them, can be an emotionally charged process. Many parents grapple with feelings of guilt, fear, and sadness when contemplating this future. It's important to recognize that these feelings are natural, but proactive planning can alleviate some of this emotional burden.

Coming to Terms with the Future

- **Acceptance**: The first step in preparing for your child's life after you is accepting that future planning is necessary, regardless of how difficult it may be. Without proper planning, your child may face unnecessary financial or legal challenges, or they may not receive the care you envisioned.

- **Seeking Support**: Many parents find that discussing their concerns with a therapist, counselor, or support group can help alleviate some of the emotional burden associated with future planning. Organizations like **The Compassionate Friends** and **Family Voices** offer counseling and peer support programs that help parents navigate these discussions.

### Choosing a Long-Term Caregiver or Guardian

One of the most important decisions you will make is selecting a long-term caregiver or guardian for your child. This individual will be responsible for making critical decisions about your child's healthcare, financial matters, and living arrangements after you are no longer able to do so.

Identifying the Right Guardian

When choosing a guardian, consider the following factors:

1. **Willingness and Capacity to Care**: Ensure that the person you select is not only willing to take on this responsibility but is also capable of doing so. Discuss the reality of caring for your child in terms of time commitment, physical care, and emotional resilience. Make sure they fully understand what will be required of them, especially if your child's condition necessitates specialized care.

2. **Compatibility**: Consider whether the potential guardian shares your values and beliefs when it comes to medical decisions, quality of life, and how you wish for your child to be raised. It's also important to consider the guardian's ability to adapt to your child's specific

emotional, physical, and developmental needs.

3. **Stability**: Choose someone who is financially stable and able to take on the financial responsibilities of guardianship, especially if your child will require lifelong care. This person should ideally have a stable living situation and be in a position to provide a secure and loving home for your child.

## Naming a Successor Guardian

It's essential to name a successor guardian in your legal documents in case the primary guardian is unable to fulfill their duties for any reason. This provides additional protection for your child, ensuring there is always someone legally responsible for their care. Successor guardianship offers peace of mind that your child's future will be in capable hands.

## Discussing the Decision with Potential Guardians

Once you have identified a potential guardian, have an honest conversation with them about the responsibilities involved and ensure they are fully prepared for the role. Provide them with comprehensive information about your child's condition, including their current treatment plans, therapies, medications, and long-term care needs. It's important to regularly revisit this conversation over time, especially if your child's condition or needs evolve.

## Estate Planning for Children with Special Needs

Estate planning is a critical part of ensuring your child's future financial security. This process involves more than just drafting a will—it encompasses creating legal structures like **Special Needs Trusts (SNTs)** and powers of attorney that ensure your child's ongoing care while protecting their access to public benefits.

**Wills and Estate Planning Basics**

In your will, you'll specify how your assets will be distributed and name a guardian for your child. However, wills alone are often insufficient for families of children with rare diseases, as leaving assets directly to your child can affect their eligibility for Medicaid or Supplemental Security Income (SSI). To prevent this, many parents choose to establish a special needs trust.

### Powers of Attorney and Healthcare Proxies

In addition to establishing trusts and wills, consider creating a **durable power of attorney** and a **healthcare proxy** for your child. A durable power of attorney allows a trusted individual to manage your child's financial affairs if they are unable to do so, while a healthcare proxy designates someone to make medical decisions on their behalf. These legal tools ensure that your child's interests are protected, even if they lack the capacity to make decisions themselves.

### Housing and Long-Term Care Options

As your child ages, their housing and care needs may change. Many parents choose to keep their child at home with the help of in-home care services, but there may come a time when residential care or group housing becomes a more viable option. Planning for this eventuality is crucial, as it ensures that your child will always have a safe, supportive living environment.

In-Home Care Options

For families who wish to keep their child at home for as long as possible, in-home care services can provide essential support. These services include:

1. **Home Health Aides**: Trained professionals who assist with daily living activities such as bathing, dressing, feeding, and medication management. Home health aides can provide a much-needed respite for family

caregivers.

2. **Nursing Services**: If your child requires medical care at home, nursing services may be available through Medicaid or private insurance. This includes skilled nursing care, such as administering medications, monitoring health conditions, or providing physical therapy.

## Residential Care Options

When in-home care is no longer feasible, there are residential care options that cater specifically to individuals with disabilities:

1. **Group Homes**: Group homes provide a supportive, community-based living environment for individuals with disabilities. These homes typically accommodate several residents who share a common space and receive 24-hour care from trained staff. Group homes focus on promoting independence while providing necessary medical and daily living assistance.

2. **Assisted Living Facilities**: Some assisted living facilities cater specifically to individuals with disabilities, offering more intensive medical care and support services than group homes. These facilities often have specialized programs for individuals with developmental or physical disabilities, including therapies, social activities, and personalized care plans.

3. **Long-Term Care Facilities**: For individuals who require constant medical supervision, long-term care facilities (nursing homes or specialized care centers) may be necessary. These facilities provide round-the-clock care, including nursing services, therapy, and medical treatment.

## Assessing Care Options

When choosing a long-term care or residential facility, it's essential to conduct thorough research. Visit potential homes, speak with staff, and ask about their experience with rare conditions similar to your child's. Consider the following factors when evaluating care options:

1. **Level of Care**: Does the facility provide the level of medical care your child needs, and do they have trained staff familiar with your child's condition?

2. **Personalized Care Plans**: How does the facility develop and implement personalized care plans? Are they flexible and adaptable as your child's needs change?

3. **Community and Socialization**: Does the facility promote community engagement, offer social activities, and encourage residents to form relationships with peers?

## Advocacy and Legacy Planning

As you plan for the future, consider leaving a legacy that reflects your values and helps continue the advocacy work you've done for your child. Many parents choose to support rare disease organizations or research initiatives as part of their legacy, helping to improve the lives of future generations affected by rare diseases.

As part of preparing for your child's future, you may also want to consider leaving behind a legacy that continues to make a positive impact on the rare disease community. Beyond securing financial and medical plans, advocacy and legacy planning provide ways to support research and resources for others who will walk a similar path in the future. This section focuses on how you can incorporate advocacy and legacy work into your long-term plans, creating a lasting influence in areas that have touched your life.

## Supporting Research and Advocacy Initiatives

Advocating for rare diseases doesn't have to stop after your child's immediate needs are met. Many families feel a strong pull to contribute to the broader community of those affected by their child's condition. Legacy planning can include efforts to support research, advance awareness campaigns, or contribute to nonprofit organizations that are working to find better treatments and improve quality of life for individuals with rare diseases.

1. **Create a Charitable Foundation**: Some families establish charitable foundations in their child's name to support rare disease research, advocacy, or provide financial aid to other families. Foundations can raise awareness of a specific condition and fund research efforts that focus on developing treatments or cures. By creating a foundation, you can leave a lasting mark on the future of healthcare for others facing similar challenges.

   - Example: The **Cystic Fibrosis Foundation** has raised significant funds for research and has been instrumental in the development of new treatments for cystic fibrosis. Starting a similar initiative for your child's rare condition can be a meaningful way to contribute to ongoing medical advancements.

2. **Contribute to Existing Organizations**: If establishing a foundation feels too ambitious, consider leaving a financial donation or creating a memorial fund within an established nonprofit organization. Organizations like **NORD (National Organization for Rare Disorders)** or **Global Genes** already have the infrastructure in place to channel donations toward research, family support, and advocacy. You could designate your donation to fund specific initiatives, such as research grants or patient assistance programs.

3. **Advocacy Through Legislation**: Advocacy efforts can also take the form of legislative support for rare disease

initiatives. By advocating for changes in healthcare policy—such as pushing for expanded insurance coverage, increased research funding, or rare disease registries—you can ensure that future generations benefit from improved medical resources. You may want to consider including advocacy goals in your legacy planning by working with organizations like **EveryLife Foundation** or **Rare Disease Legislative Advocates (RDLA)**, which focus on policy improvements and legislative change in rare disease healthcare.

### Incorporating Charitable Contributions in Estate Planning

Many families choose to include charitable contributions in their estate planning as a way of supporting research or helping other families coping with similar challenges. This can be done in a few ways:

1. **Charitable Trusts**: Establish a **charitable remainder trust** or **charitable lead trust** that donates part of your estate to a nonprofit organization while still providing income to your family members or designated heirs.

2. **Bequests**: Leave a portion of your estate or life insurance payout to a charitable organization. Bequests can be earmarked for specific purposes, such as funding a rare disease research grant, providing family financial aid, or supporting community outreach programs.

3. **Donor-Advised Funds**: A **donor-advised fund (DAF)** allows you to contribute assets to a fund that grows tax-free over time, with the eventual goal of distributing those funds to charitable organizations. You can work with a financial advisor to create a DAF that supports rare disease research, family advocacy, or other causes related to your child's condition.

## Honoring Your Child's Legacy

In addition to financial and advocacy planning, many families find comfort in creating tangible ways to honor their child's legacy. This can take the form of:

- **Memorial Scholarships**: Establish a scholarship fund in your child's name to support students studying fields related to rare disease research or healthcare. Scholarships can also be directed toward students with disabilities or those overcoming challenges similar to your child's.

- **Awareness Campaigns**: Organize awareness events, such as annual walks, runs, or fundraising galas that bring attention to your child's condition and raise funds for research and advocacy.

- **Written or Video Memorials**: Some families create written memoirs, blogs, or video documentaries that share their child's journey with the world. These memorials can offer support and encouragement to others going through similar experiences, while also raising awareness for rare diseases.

## Life Insurance: Protecting Your Child's Financial Future

While estate planning and trusts protect your child's long-term needs, **life insurance** is another vital tool to ensure they are financially secure. In this section, we explore how life insurance policies can be structured to support your child after your death.

Choosing the Right Life Insurance Policy

1. **Term Life Insurance**: Term life insurance provides coverage for a specific period—usually 10, 20, or 30 years—and is a cost-effective way to ensure financial security during the years your child is most dependent on you. A term policy can provide a significant death

benefit that goes directly into a special needs trust (SNT) or ABLE account to cover medical and daily living expenses.

2. **Whole Life Insurance**: Whole life insurance provides permanent coverage and builds cash value over time. This policy can serve as a long-term safety net for your child, especially if their condition requires lifelong care. The death benefit can be directed to a special needs trust, ensuring that the funds are used to support your child without affecting their eligibility for Medicaid or SSI.

3. **Universal Life Insurance**: Similar to whole life insurance, **universal life insurance** offers lifelong coverage, but with flexible premiums and the ability to adjust the death benefit as needed. The cash value of the policy can be used to supplement your child's financial needs while you are alive, or it can be allocated to their care after you pass.

## Designating a Beneficiary

When setting up a life insurance policy for your child with a rare disease, it's important to designate a special needs trust (SNT) as the **primary beneficiary** rather than leaving the funds directly to your child. Direct inheritance of life insurance proceeds can disqualify your child from critical government benefits like Medicaid and SSI, as receiving a large sum of money would exceed the asset limits for these programs. By naming the trust as the beneficiary, you can ensure that the funds are used to enhance your child's quality of life without affecting their benefits.

Planning for your child's future—particularly in a world without you—is one of the most challenging aspects of raising a child with a rare disease. However, by taking proactive steps to select a long-term caregiver, establish financial safeguards like special needs trusts, and create a legacy that supports research and advocacy, you can provide your child with the security they need.

From securing life insurance and organizing legal documents to supporting research and advocacy, every step of future planning offers peace of mind for you and ensures your child will be well cared for in the years to come. The key to success is to begin planning early, revisit your plans regularly, and engage with financial, legal, and medical professionals who specialize in supporting families of children with special needs.

By focusing on these areas, you can build a robust framework that not only protects your child's health and well-being but also leaves a lasting legacy for future generations affected by rare diseases.

# CHAPTER 8: NAVIGATING GRIEF AND LOSS—COPING WITH THE UNTHINKABLE

Caring for a child with a rare condition often comes with the painful knowledge that their life might be shortened by their illness. For some families, this devastating reality culminates in the loss of their child, an unimaginable tragedy. In this chapter, we will explore the unique and complex nature of grief associated with losing a child, how to navigate this grief, and the available resources to help families cope. Whether your child's condition is terminal or their loss was sudden and unexpected, grief is a profoundly personal journey. Understanding and finding support during this process is crucial to long-term healing.

## The Nature of Grief After Losing a Child

Losing a child is often described as one of the most painful experiences a person can endure. Unlike other forms of grief, the death of a child can feel unnatural and shattering to the core. Parents may not only grieve the loss of their child but also the future they had hoped for. They may mourn milestones their child will never reach—graduations, weddings, or simply growing up. This kind of grief, particularly when linked to a rare disease, can be layered with years of anticipatory grief, guilt, or even relief that the child is no longer suffering.

Types of Grief in Parental Loss

1. **Anticipatory Grief**: Parents of children with terminal conditions often experience **anticipatory grief**—the

grief that begins even before the child passes. This grief, which can span months or years, includes feelings of fear, sadness, and anxiety as parents prepare for the loss of their child. While difficult, anticipatory grief can also provide parents the opportunity to create memories and say meaningful goodbyes.

2. **Acute Grief**: After the loss, many parents experience **acute grief**—the intense wave of emotional pain that hits immediately following their child's death. This grief is often accompanied by shock, disbelief, and numbness, even when the death was expected.

3. **Complicated Grief**: For some, grief may persist far longer and more intensely than expected, becoming **complicated grief**. Parents who struggle to return to their daily lives, isolate themselves from others, or feel an overwhelming sense of hopelessness may need additional support to process their grief healthily.

4. **Disenfranchised Grief**: Parents whose children have had rare or chronic conditions may experience **disenfranchised grief**, where their loss is not fully recognized or supported by society. Because the child's death may be seen as "expected," others may not acknowledge the depth of the parent's grief, leading to feelings of isolation.

## The Process of Grieving

The **stages of grief**—denial, anger, bargaining, depression, and acceptance—are well-known, but it is important to understand that grief is not a linear process. Parents may cycle through these stages repeatedly or in different orders. Everyone's grief journey is unique, and the process of healing takes time, often lasting far longer than society expects. Below are key insights into each stage of grief and how parents might navigate them:

1. **Denial**: Denial is often the brain's way of cushioning

the blow of overwhelming news. Even after a prolonged illness, parents may struggle to believe that their child is truly gone. This disbelief can provide temporary emotional protection, allowing them to process their grief at a slower pace.

2. **Anger**: It is common to feel anger after losing a child, often directed at the healthcare system, medical professionals, or even oneself. Parents may feel that life is profoundly unfair or that they could have done something differently to prevent their child's death. Acknowledging and expressing this anger is an important part of the grieving process.

3. **Bargaining**: Parents may find themselves bargaining with fate or dwelling on "what if" scenarios. This can manifest as feelings of guilt—wondering if they missed early signs of illness or if a different course of treatment would have changed the outcome.

4. **Depression**: As the reality of the loss sets in, parents may experience profound sadness, withdrawal from social activities, and a feeling of emptiness. While painful, this stage is necessary for fully processing the loss. Some parents may need professional support to cope with feelings of depression, especially if it becomes debilitating.

5. **Acceptance**: Acceptance does not mean "getting over" the loss of a child but rather finding a way to move forward with life while still carrying the memory of the child. Acceptance is often the result of a long and ongoing process that allows parents to find meaning in life again.

**Finding Support After Loss**

No one should have to navigate the loss of a child alone. Support from family, friends, counselors, and community groups can help parents cope with their grief and find ways to heal over time. Below are some key resources and strategies for finding support:

Grief Counseling

- **Grief counselors** specialize in helping individuals process their emotions following a significant loss. For parents, this may include addressing feelings of guilt, anger, or prolonged sadness. Therapists often use techniques like **cognitive-behavioral therapy (CBT)** or **trauma-informed therapy** to help parents reframe negative thoughts and manage their grief in a healthy way.

- **Family therapy** can also be beneficial, especially if surviving siblings or extended family members are struggling to cope with the loss. Family therapy provides a space for everyone to express their emotions and work through the grieving process together.

Support Groups

- **The Compassionate Friends** is one of the largest organizations providing support to parents who have lost a child. They offer both in-person and virtual support groups, allowing parents to connect with others who are experiencing similar grief.

- **GriefShare** is a Christian-based grief support program that offers groups specifically for those grieving the loss of a loved one. They provide tools, resources, and a sense of community during the grieving process.

- **Bereaved Parents of the USA**: This organization offers both local chapters and national resources for parents grieving the loss of a child. They also provide online forums and newsletters that allow parents to share their experiences and support each other.

Online Support Communities

- **The Mighty** and **RareConnect** offer online communities where families affected by rare diseases can connect with others facing similar challenges. These platforms offer emotional support, advice, and a sense of solidarity among parents who understand the unique pain of losing a child to a rare disease.

## Caring for Yourself While Grieving

Grief can take a significant toll on both physical and mental health. It is important for parents to prioritize self-care during this time, even if it feels impossible. Grief is exhausting, and many parents neglect their own well-being while trying to cope with the loss. Below are strategies for taking care of yourself while grieving:

1. **Give Yourself Permission to Feel**: Allow yourself to feel the full range of emotions, from sadness to anger to confusion. Suppressing grief can make the healing process longer and more difficult.

2. **Rest and Nutrition**: Grief is physically exhausting, and many parents find that their sleep patterns are disrupted after losing a child. Try to maintain a regular sleep schedule and eat nutritious meals, even if your appetite is low. Taking care of your physical body can help you manage the emotional strain.

3. **Exercise**: Light exercise, such as walking, yoga, or swimming, can help relieve some of the physical tension caused by grief. Physical activity also releases endorphins, which can improve mood and energy levels.

4. **Seek Professional Help**: If you find that your grief is preventing you from functioning in your daily life or if feelings of hopelessness persist for an extended period, it may be helpful to seek professional therapy. There is

no shame in asking for help when you need it.

## Coping with the Loss of a Sibling

It's not just parents who grieve the loss of a child—siblings often experience intense feelings of loss, too. Children and teenagers may have difficulty processing their emotions and may feel isolated if they don't have the vocabulary to express their grief.

Helping Siblings Process the Loss

1. **Open Dialogue**: Encourage open conversations with surviving siblings. Answer their questions honestly and provide explanations that are age-appropriate. Let them know that it's okay to feel sad, confused, or even angry.

2. **Involvement in Memorials**: Involving siblings in memorial services or remembrance activities, such as creating a memory box or participating in a memorial walk, can help them process their grief and say goodbye in their own way.

3. **Support Groups for Children**: Many grief support organizations offer specialized support for children who have lost a sibling. **The Dougy Center** provides resources and support for grieving children, offering both in-person and online programs [24†source] .

## Finding Meaning After Loss

Many parents find that creating a legacy in their child's name helps them cope with their grief and gives them a sense of purpose. For some, this may involve advocacy, raising awareness about their child's condition, or creating a memorial fund to support rare disease research.

Creating a Legacy

- **Scholarships and Memorial Funds**: Some families establish scholarships in their child's name to support education in areas like healthcare, research, or social work.

- **Advocacy for Rare Diseases**: Parents can honor their child's legacy by becoming advocates for rare disease research, awareness, or policy changes. Organizations like **Global Genes** and **NORD** provide platforms for parents to share their stories and advocate for better care and resources for rare diseases.

When caring for a child with a rare condition, thoughts about the future may be dominated by the hope of better treatments, improved care, and shared milestones. However, for some families, the painful reality of losing a child becomes inevitable. Whether the loss is anticipated due to the progressive nature of a terminal illness or it happens unexpectedly, parents and caregivers are faced with the unimaginable. This chapter explores the journey of grief and loss, providing insight into how families can cope, find support, and navigate the emotional, mental, and practical challenges that arise when a child passes away.

## The Unique Nature of Parental Grief

Grieving the loss of a child is one of the most profound and intense forms of grief. Unlike other losses, the death of a child feels unnatural, and many parents find themselves mourning not only their child's life but also the future they had imagined for them. This complex grief often combines elements of anticipatory grief, acute grief, and even relief if the child's life had been marked by immense suffering. Grief for parents is not just about saying goodbye but also reconciling with the idea that their child's story will never reach the milestones they once hoped for.

## Anticipatory Grief

Parents of children with terminal illnesses often experience **anticipatory grief**, which begins long before their child passes. This form of grief can be emotionally taxing as parents grapple with the knowledge that their child's life may be cut short. Anticipatory grief is a blend of preparing emotionally for the inevitable and trying to remain present for their child's current needs. It allows some parents the opportunity to say goodbye and create meaningful memories during their child's final days, though it doesn't lessen the pain when the loss occurs.

### Acute Grief

The period immediately following the loss is marked by **acute grief**—an overwhelming wave of emotions such as shock, disbelief, and profound sadness. Even when death is anticipated, it can still feel surreal, as though it has arrived too soon. Acute grief may also involve feelings of numbness or detachment, as the mind struggles to process the finality of the loss. Many parents find that during this stage, basic tasks like eating, sleeping, or engaging in conversation become incredibly difficult.

### Complicated Grief

For some parents, grief persists far longer than anticipated and begins to interfere with daily functioning—this is known as **complicated grief**. It manifests in feelings of deep sadness, hopelessness, and an inability to move forward with life. Parents experiencing complicated grief may feel stuck, unable to see a way forward without their child. When grief becomes all-consuming, professional intervention through therapy or counseling is often necessary to guide parents toward healing.

### Disenfranchised Grief

In certain cases, parents may feel their grief is not fully recognized or validated, especially if their child's death is seen as an expected outcome due to a long-term illness. This is known as **disenfranchised grief**, where societal expectations may minimize the significance of the loss. Well-meaning friends or family members may suggest that parents should find solace in the idea that their child is "no longer suffering," but this perspective can exacerbate feelings of isolation for the grieving parents. Each child's life, no matter how brief or filled with challenges, is worth mourning.

## Emotional and Psychological Healing After Loss

The grieving process is deeply personal, and no two parents experience it the same way. While some may feel the need to retreat and grieve in solitude, others may seek out community and connection to share their loss. It's essential to acknowledge that grief is a process, not a singular event, and it can last months, years, or even a lifetime. Understanding that emotional healing happens in waves—sometimes with progress, and other times with setbacks—can help parents navigate this difficult journey.

## The Nonlinear Nature of Grief

Grief does not follow a clear timeline or set of stages. While the classic **five stages of grief**—denial, anger, bargaining, depression, and acceptance—are commonly referenced, most parents find themselves moving between these stages in a non-linear fashion. Grief may change day-to-day, and parents might experience multiple emotions simultaneously or return to feelings they thought had been resolved. This emotional complexity is normal and should be embraced as part of the healing process.

## Support Systems for Grieving Parents

Grief is intensely personal, but parents should know that they don't have to go through it alone. Support systems—whether through family, friends, professional counselors, or peer support groups—are essential for emotional healing.

- **Grief Counseling**: Working with a grief counselor can provide parents with the tools to process their emotions and find healthy ways to cope. Professional therapists specializing in trauma or bereavement often use techniques such as **cognitive-behavioral therapy (CBT)** or **acceptance and commitment therapy (ACT)** to help parents manage their grief.

- **Support Groups**: Joining a support group for parents who have lost a child can provide a sense of community and shared understanding. Organizations like **The Compassionate Friends** and **Bereaved Parents of the USA** offer both local and online support groups, where parents can talk about their grief and find comfort in knowing they are not alone.

- **Journaling and Creative Expression**: Some parents find solace in writing about their grief or expressing their emotions through art, music, or other creative outlets. Journaling allows for private reflection, while creative projects can offer a sense of purpose during a time of profound loss.

### The Impact of Grief on Siblings and Family Dynamics

While parents bear the brunt of grief after losing a child, the impact of the loss is felt throughout the entire family. Siblings often experience grief in unique ways, and their emotional needs may be overlooked as parents navigate their own sorrow. It's important to provide support for siblings and other family members, ensuring that everyone has the opportunity to express their feelings and receive the help they need.

Grieving the loss of a child is an excruciating and life-altering experience. There is no right or wrong way to grieve, and the path to healing is unique for every parent. By acknowledging the complexity of grief, seeking support from others, and finding ways to honor your child's memory, families can gradually learn to live with their loss while cherishing the time they had with their child.

While the pain of losing a child never fully disappears, many parents find comfort and purpose through memorial projects, advocacy, or simply sharing their child's story. Grief, in its many forms, becomes a part of the fabric of their lives—woven into their identity as parents who loved, lost, and continue to honor their child's legacy.

## *CHAPTER 9: ADVOCACY AND FINDING YOUR VOICE —STANDING UP FOR YOUR CHILD AND COMMUNITY*

Advocating for a child with a rare disease is one of the most important roles a parent or caregiver can undertake. Advocacy involves navigating complex healthcare systems, fighting for educational rights, raising awareness, and influencing policies that impact both your child and the broader rare disease community. This chapter delves into how parents can become effective advocates, offering strategies for engaging with healthcare providers, schools, insurance companies, and government policymakers. It also highlights the power of community advocacy and how individual voices can spark collective change.

### The Importance of Advocacy in Rare Diseases

Advocacy is essential in rare diseases because the very nature of these conditions often means that awareness, resources, and expertise are limited. Many healthcare providers, educators, and policymakers may not be familiar with your child's specific condition, making it crucial for you to step in as their voice. Advocacy involves much more than simply asking for better care or support; it's about educating those around you, navigating complex bureaucracies, and, most importantly, ensuring that your child's needs are met—whether that's access to proper healthcare, educational accommodations, or financial support.

Why Advocacy is Different for Rare Diseases

1. **Lack of Awareness**: Unlike common conditions, rare diseases are not as widely known, even among medical professionals. Many families report encountering healthcare providers who are unfamiliar with their child's diagnosis, leading to misdiagnoses, delays in treatment, or suboptimal care. Advocating for your child often means becoming an expert on their condition and educating those around you about the specific needs and challenges your child faces.

2. **Limited Resources**: The rarity of these conditions often means that there are fewer resources—whether it's in terms of research, clinical trials, or specialized care. Many parents must push for access to these limited resources, whether it's securing a spot in a specialized treatment program or finding a provider who is willing to work with a complex case.

3. **Insurance and Coverage Issues**: Treatments for rare diseases can be expensive, and insurance companies may deny coverage for what they deem experimental treatments or therapies. Advocacy often means filing appeals and pushing back against insurance denials, making a case for why these treatments are essential for your child's quality of life.

## Becoming an Advocate in the Healthcare System

Navigating the healthcare system is one of the most critical areas where advocacy comes into play. As a parent, you are your child's primary advocate when it comes to their medical care. You will need to coordinate between specialists, ensure that your child receives timely and appropriate treatments, and sometimes push for second opinions or experimental treatments. The following are key strategies for becoming an effective medical advocate.

Steps to Effective Medical Advocacy

1. **Educate Yourself**: The first step in medical advocacy is becoming as informed as possible about your child's condition. This includes researching the disease, understanding its progression, and staying up to date with the latest treatment options. Patient advocacy groups like **Global Genes** or the **National Organization for Rare Disorders (NORD)** provide invaluable resources for learning more about rare diseases, connecting with experts, and finding treatment options.

2. **Build a Medical Team**: Many rare diseases require multidisciplinary care, involving specialists in fields like neurology, genetics, cardiology, or immunology. It's important to build a team of doctors who communicate well with each other and understand your child's needs. Advocating for coordinated care ensures that your child's treatment is holistic and that no aspect of their condition is overlooked.

3. **Document Everything**: Keeping meticulous records is essential when advocating for your child's healthcare. Create a medical binder that includes all test results, diagnoses, treatment plans, and correspondence with doctors. This not only helps you stay organized but also provides you with the necessary information to refer to when pushing for certain treatments or second opinions.

4. **Don't Be Afraid to Seek Second Opinions**: In the world of rare diseases, it's not uncommon for parents to seek second, third, or even fourth opinions. Specialists may have different approaches to treatment, and it's important to feel confident that your child is receiving the best possible care. Many renowned hospitals, like **Boston Children's Hospital**, **Cleveland Clinic**, and the **Mayo Clinic**, offer second opinion services, which can

help guide you to the most effective treatment options.

5. **Communicate Assertively**: Healthcare providers are experts in their fields, but you are the expert on your child. Don't be afraid to ask questions, request additional tests, or push for alternative treatment plans. Clear, assertive communication is key when advocating for your child's medical care. If necessary, you can also enlist the help of a patient advocate or care coordinator who can assist with navigating the complexities of healthcare systems.

## Advocating with Insurance Companies

Health insurance plays a major role in determining what treatments and therapies your child can access. Unfortunately, it's not uncommon for insurance companies to deny coverage for treatments they deem unnecessary or experimental—particularly in the realm of rare diseases. Advocacy often means learning how to navigate the insurance process, filing appeals, and fighting for your child's right to access life-saving treatments.

### Appealing Denied Claims

If your insurance company denies a claim for a necessary treatment, it's important to file an appeal as soon as possible. Here's how to approach this process:

1. **Understand the Denial**: Request a written explanation from the insurance company as to why the claim was denied. This will often include specific reasons, such as the treatment being considered experimental or not medically necessary.

2. **Gather Documentation**: Work with your child's healthcare providers to gather documentation supporting the need for the treatment. This could include letters from specialists, medical records,

or scientific research showing the treatment's effectiveness.

3. **Submit a Formal Appeal**: Insurance companies have a formal appeals process that typically involves submitting a written appeal along with supporting documentation. Be sure to include any letters from doctors and detailed explanations of why the treatment is necessary for your child's health.

4. **Request an Independent Review**: If the appeal is denied, you have the right to request an independent external review. In this process, a third-party reviewer will assess whether the insurance company's decision to deny the treatment was justified. Many parents find success in getting treatments approved through this review process.

## Community and Legislative Advocacy

While personal advocacy is essential, many families also choose to engage in **community and legislative advocacy** to support broader change. Whether it's raising awareness about rare diseases, pushing for increased research funding, or fighting for policy changes that improve access to care, community advocacy can have a significant impact.

## Raising Awareness

Raising awareness about rare diseases is a powerful form of advocacy. Whether it's through social media, local events, or national campaigns, parents and caregivers can help shed light on the challenges of living with rare diseases. Organizations like **Rare Disease Day**, celebrated annually on the last day of February, encourage families to share their stories and advocate for greater public awareness.

## Advocating for Policy Change

Legislative advocacy is another key area where parents can make a difference. By working with advocacy organizations like the **EveryLife Foundation for Rare Diseases**, parents can push for policy changes that improve access to care, increase funding for research, and ensure that rare disease patients are represented in healthcare policy discussions. Advocacy efforts might include meeting with legislators, participating in awareness campaigns, or writing to government officials to share personal stories and advocate for changes in healthcare laws.

Becoming an advocate for your child with a rare disease is an ongoing journey that spans the healthcare system, educational institutions, insurance companies, and legislative forums. It involves raising your voice to ensure that your child receives the best possible care, while also contributing to the larger rare disease community. Advocacy is a powerful tool for influencing change, whether on a personal level—ensuring your child's immediate needs are met—or on a societal level, fighting for better research funding, legislative reforms, and wider awareness of rare conditions.

By educating yourself, building strong relationships with healthcare providers, staying organized, and assertively pursuing necessary treatments and accommodations, you can be a formidable advocate for your child. Alongside individual efforts, community and legislative advocacy give you the opportunity to create lasting changes that benefit all families affected by rare diseases.

As you continue on this path, remember that advocacy is a collaborative effort, and you are not alone. Countless organizations, support groups, and other parents are walking this same road, working together to build a more inclusive and informed society where every child has access to the care and support they need.

# CHAPTER 10: CULTIVATING RESILIENCE—SUSTAINING HOPE IN THE FACE OF CHALLENGES

Raising a child with a rare condition is a long and often arduous journey, filled with emotional, financial, and physical challenges. However, one of the key elements that help families navigate these difficulties is resilience. Resilience isn't just about surviving adversity; it's about finding ways to adapt, grow, and even thrive despite the obstacles. In this chapter, we will explore what resilience looks like in the context of rare disease caregiving, how to build and sustain it, and how it can transform both the caregiver and child's experiences.

## Understanding Resilience

Resilience is often defined as the ability to bounce back from hardship, but in the context of rare diseases, it goes beyond merely returning to a previous state of well-being. Resilience involves growth, learning, and adapting to new realities. For parents of children with rare diseases, resilience manifests as the capacity to continually face overwhelming challenges—such as navigating complex medical systems, handling emotional strain, and balancing caregiving with personal and professional obligations —while maintaining hope and seeking solutions.

Emotional and Psychological Resilience

The emotional toll of caring for a child with a rare condition is significant. Parents often deal with chronic stress, anxiety about their child's future, and the grief that comes with watching a child struggle. Building emotional resilience means developing strategies to manage these emotions while staying focused on long-term goals for your child's care.

1. **Emotional Flexibility**: Resilient parents are able to shift their emotional responses based on the situation. For example, they may practice **mindfulness** techniques to stay present and avoid getting overwhelmed by fear of the future. Mindfulness can help caregivers focus on the present moment, reducing anxiety and stress by shifting attention away from worst-case scenarios and onto actionable tasks in the here and now.

2. **Self-Compassion**: Many parents feel a strong sense of guilt when they cannot "fix" their child's condition or when they experience burnout. Resilience involves recognizing the limits of what one person can control and practicing self-compassion. Studies have shown that self-compassion—treating yourself with the same kindness you would offer to a friend—can significantly reduce caregiver stress.

3. **Finding Meaning**: A critical element of emotional resilience is finding meaning in the caregiving journey. Whether through advocacy, community involvement, or simply reflecting on the love and connection shared with their child, many parents find that meaning helps them cope with the hardships of caregiving. **Viktor Frankl's** theory of meaning-making, often referred to as **logotherapy**, suggests that when individuals find purpose in suffering, they are better able to endure it.

### Building Physical and Mental Endurance

Resilience isn't just psychological—physical and mental endurance are essential aspects of long-term caregiving. Many caregivers report experiencing physical exhaustion and burnout due to the constant demands of caring for a child with a rare disease. Learning to manage your physical health while caring for someone else is crucial in sustaining resilience.

The Importance of Physical Self-Care

1. **Regular Exercise**: Incorporating exercise into your daily routine can boost both physical and emotional resilience. Exercise is not only a way to maintain physical strength for caregiving tasks, but it also releases endorphins, which can improve mood and reduce feelings of stress or anxiety. Simple activities such as walking, stretching, or practicing yoga can make a significant difference.

2. **Adequate Sleep**: Sleep deprivation is common among caregivers, particularly those caring for children who require nighttime monitoring or frequent interventions. However, chronic sleep deprivation can weaken immune function, exacerbate emotional stress, and increase the risk of burnout. Strategies such as taking shifts with a partner, utilizing respite care, or scheduling naps throughout the day can help improve sleep quality.

3. **Nutrition and Hydration**: Caregivers often neglect their own nutrition as they prioritize the needs of their child. However, maintaining a balanced diet rich in fruits, vegetables, and lean proteins can provide the energy and mental clarity necessary to face daily challenges. Staying hydrated is also key, as dehydration can lead to fatigue, headaches, and irritability, further exacerbating stress.

**Cognitive Resilience: Managing Mental Fatigue**

Cognitive resilience refers to the ability to stay focused, organized, and mentally sharp even in the face of overwhelming demands. Caregivers are often required to manage complex medical schedules, juggle appointments, and keep track of medications, all while handling everyday household responsibilities. **Mental fatigue** is a common issue, but strategies exist to bolster cognitive resilience:

1. **Delegation**: Learning to delegate tasks—whether to other family members, friends, or healthcare professionals—can alleviate some of the cognitive load that caregivers bear. Delegating allows caregivers to focus on essential tasks and reduce the mental strain that comes from trying to manage everything on their own.

2. **Time Management Tools**: Utilizing time management tools such as calendars, to-do lists, and reminder apps can help caregivers stay organized and reduce the mental energy required to keep track of tasks. Tools like **Google Calendar**, **Trello**, or **CareZone** (which is specifically designed for managing healthcare needs) allow for effective scheduling and communication with other caregivers or family members.

3. **Mindfulness and Meditation**: Regular meditation or mindfulness practices can improve focus, reduce stress, and increase cognitive clarity. Even five to ten minutes of meditation each day can help reframe stressful situations and prevent burnout. Apps like **Headspace** or **Calm** offer guided meditation sessions tailored to reducing stress and improving mental resilience.

### The Role of Community in Building Resilience

While resilience is often seen as a personal quality, community support plays a critical role in helping caregivers sustain their strength. The concept of **community resilience** involves drawing on collective resources, knowledge, and emotional support from others who understand your situation. For families dealing with rare diseases, connecting with a network of people facing similar challenges can provide a lifeline during difficult times.

Support Groups and Online Communities

1. **Peer Support Groups**: Joining a support group—either in person or online—allows parents and caregivers to share experiences, offer advice, and provide emotional support to one another. Organizations like **Global Genes**, **The Mighty**, and **NORD** offer platforms for caregivers to connect with others who understand the unique challenges of raising a child with a rare condition.

2. **Respite Care**: One of the most tangible forms of community support is **respite care**—temporary care provided by someone else to give the primary caregiver a break. Respite care can be offered through family, friends, or professional services. Programs like **ARCH National Respite Network** connect families to respite care resources, providing caregivers with the time they need to rest and recharge.

3. **Advocacy Communities**: Being part of an advocacy group not only provides emotional support but also offers a sense of purpose. Working together to raise awareness for rare diseases, secure research funding, or improve healthcare policies can give caregivers a collective mission that sustains their resilience. Many parents find strength and encouragement by participating in events like **Rare Disease Day**, where they can share their stories and advocate for better care and resources.

**Resilience and Adaptability in Managing Medical Challenges**

The medical aspect of caring for a child with a rare disease often requires families to be adaptable in the face of changing circumstances. Treatments may not work as expected, new symptoms may arise, and there may be moments when all plans need to change suddenly. Being flexible and resilient in the face of medical challenges is crucial.

Navigating Changing Treatment Plans

1. **Seeking Second Opinions**: As new treatments or therapies become available, it's important for families to remain open to changing medical plans. Seeking second or third opinions from specialists, particularly when treatments seem ineffective or stalled, is an essential aspect of medical resilience. Consulting with top medical institutions like **Mayo Clinic** or **Cleveland Clinic**, which have rare disease programs, can provide new insights or alternative approaches.

2. **Managing Setbacks**: Many rare diseases are unpredictable, and there may be setbacks in your child's health despite the best efforts of medical teams. Resilience in this context means understanding that progress is not always linear. Families who have developed resilience tend to focus on small victories and remain hopeful even when things don't go as planned.

3. **Staying Informed**: One key to medical resilience is staying informed about the latest advancements in treatments, therapies, and research related to your child's condition. This includes joining clinical trials if appropriate and keeping up with research being conducted through organizations like the **National Institutes of Health (NIH)** or **NORD**.

**Long-Term Resilience: Thinking About the Future**

For many families, building resilience means thinking about the long-term—planning not only for the immediate challenges of caring for a child with a rare condition but also for their future. This can include financial planning, legal protections, and long-term care options.

Financial Resilience

1. **Financial Planning Tools**: Managing the financial burden of rare disease care can be overwhelming. Building financial resilience means seeking out financial assistance programs, grants, and insurance plans that can offset costs. Tools like **special needs trusts** and **ABLE accounts** help families save for long-term care without jeopardizing government benefits.

2. **Life Insurance and Estate Planning**: Families need to ensure that their child will be taken care of in the event of the caregiver's death. Life insurance policies, estate planning, and the designation of a guardian are essential steps in building long-term resilience

# CHAPTER 11: THE POWER OF HOPE—FINDING LIGHT IN DIFFICULT TIMES

Raising a child with a rare condition brings with it numerous challenges, from navigating complex medical systems to dealing with emotional stress and uncertainty. However, through it all, **hope** remains one of the most essential tools for parents and caregivers. Hope is not simply a vague optimism; it's a powerful, actionable force that can sustain families through difficult times, foster resilience, and drive advocacy efforts. This chapter explores the transformative power of hope and how families can harness it to improve their child's quality of life, stay motivated, and find meaning amidst adversity.

## Understanding the Role of Hope

For many parents of children with rare diseases, hope can take on many forms. It might mean hoping for a medical breakthrough, a new treatment, or a clinical trial that could improve their child's prognosis. It can also mean finding hope in smaller, everyday victories—whether it's seeing improvement in a child's developmental milestones, getting through a difficult medical procedure, or simply experiencing moments of joy and connection with their child.

## The Science of Hope

Hope is not just an abstract feeling; it has been studied in the fields of psychology and neuroscience. **Positive psychology** research has shown that hope contributes to better mental and physical health outcomes. According to **Dr. Charles Snyder**, a prominent psychologist who developed the **Hope Theory**, hope is comprised of two key components: **agency** (the belief that you can initiate and sustain action to reach your goals) and **pathways** (the ability to develop strategies or routes to achieve those goals). This model of hope suggests that parents who are able to envision clear pathways toward helping their child—whether through medical treatments, therapies, or advocacy—are more likely to feel empowered and motivated.

Studies have shown that individuals with higher levels of hope tend to have better coping mechanisms when faced with adversity. In the context of healthcare, patients and caregivers who maintain hope are more likely to be proactive in seeking new treatments, advocating for their needs, and maintaining mental health. This concept of **action-oriented hope** encourages families to focus not only on long-term goals but also on immediate, achievable steps that lead to better outcomes.

### Harnessing Hope Through Action

Parents of children with rare diseases often find that their hope is driven by concrete actions they can take to improve their child's care and well-being. Hope can be nurtured by becoming an active participant in your child's care, whether through medical advocacy, connecting with supportive communities, or staying informed about the latest research.

Medical Advocacy as a Source of Hope

One of the most powerful ways to maintain hope is by advocating for your child within the healthcare system. Being an informed, proactive advocate allows you to take control of situations that might otherwise feel overwhelming. Some key steps include:

1. **Staying Informed**: Knowledge is a powerful tool

for maintaining hope. Keeping up with the latest research, medical advancements, and treatment options can provide families with new opportunities and avenues to explore. Organizations like **NORD (National Organization for Rare Disorders)** and **Global Genes** offer resources that help families stay informed about new clinical trials, emerging therapies, and advocacy initiatives.

2. **Clinical Trials**: For many rare diseases, there may be limited treatment options, making clinical trials a beacon of hope. Participating in clinical trials allows families to access experimental therapies that could improve their child's quality of life or slow disease progression. Websites like **ClinicalTrials.gov** provide a comprehensive database of ongoing trials, allowing families to search for trials that are specific to their child's condition.

3. **Seeking Second Opinions**: When traditional treatment paths seem limited, hope can come from seeking second opinions or consulting with specialists at top medical centers. Major institutions like **Mayo Clinic**, **Cleveland Clinic**, and **Boston Children's Hospital** offer specialized care for rare diseases and are often at the forefront of developing new treatments. Knowing that there are experts actively working on your child's condition can be incredibly reassuring.

### Connecting with Support Networks

Community plays a significant role in sustaining hope. Parents and caregivers who connect with others facing similar challenges often report feeling less isolated and more empowered. Support networks provide both emotional comfort and practical advice, helping families navigate the complexities of rare disease care.

1. **Parent Support Groups**: Joining support groups allows

parents to share their experiences, offer advice, and provide encouragement to one another. **The Mighty** and **RareConnect** are two platforms that offer online forums where families can find a sense of community and exchange information. Parents often find hope in knowing that others have walked a similar path and are available to provide guidance.

2. **Respite and Caregiver Support**: Many families find renewed hope through respite care services, which provide temporary relief from the daily demands of caregiving. Programs like the **ARCH National Respite Network** connect families with resources to help them take time for themselves. Having the opportunity to rest and recharge allows parents to return to caregiving with a renewed sense of energy and hope.

3. **Advocacy Organizations**: Many families also find hope in advocacy work, particularly when they can connect with organizations that are dedicated to raising awareness or funding research for their child's condition. Advocacy work not only offers a sense of purpose but also provides hope that future treatments, policies, and resources will improve the lives of all children with rare diseases.

### Finding Hope in Daily Life

While hope can often be driven by long-term goals like finding a cure or improving treatment options, it's also important to cultivate hope in daily life. Small victories—whether they are health improvements, new developmental milestones, or simply moments of joy—can serve as powerful reminders of the strength and resilience both parents and children possess.

### Focusing on Small Wins

For many parents, large-scale progress can seem slow or uncertain, especially in the world of rare diseases where medical advancements may take years. By focusing on small, incremental victories, families can find hope in the present moment. Some examples of small wins might include:

1. **Developmental Milestones**: Celebrating even the smallest developmental gains—whether it's a child learning a new word, making eye contact, or mastering a physical skill—can provide a sense of progress and hope for future achievements.

2. **Positive Medical Outcomes**: Even when long-term treatments are slow to take effect, smaller victories, like a successful surgery or reduced symptoms after treatment, offer tangible progress to celebrate.

3. **Moments of Joy**: Finding joy in daily interactions with your child—whether it's through laughter, playing, or simply spending time together—can provide emotional nourishment. Many parents find that taking time to appreciate these moments strengthens their emotional resilience and reinforces their sense of hope.

## Balancing Hope with Acceptance

While hope is a vital tool for coping with the challenges of rare diseases, it's important to balance hope with acceptance. Acceptance does not mean giving up on finding solutions or progress; rather, it means coming to terms with the realities of your child's condition and focusing on what can be done to improve their quality of life. Acceptance and hope are not mutually exclusive but can coexist in a way that allows families to remain realistic while still striving for better outcomes.

## Hope and Realism

Maintaining hope in the face of difficult medical realities can sometimes feel like walking a fine line between optimism and realism. Resilient families find ways to balance these two perspectives by staying hopeful for new treatments or improvements while also acknowledging the current limitations of their child's condition. Some strategies for balancing hope and realism include:

1. **Setting Realistic Goals**: While it's important to hope for breakthroughs or cures, it's equally important to set realistic, achievable goals for your child's care. This might mean focusing on improving your child's quality of life through physical therapy, speech therapy, or pain management while remaining open to future advancements.

2. **Practicing Gratitude**: Gratitude and hope often go hand in hand. By focusing on the things that are going well —whether it's a caring medical team, supportive friends and family, or small health improvements—parents can cultivate a sense of gratitude that reinforces their hope for the future.

### The Power of Faith and Spirituality

For many families, hope is deeply intertwined with faith and spirituality. Spiritual practices, prayer, or religious communities can provide a profound sense of comfort and hope in times of uncertainty. Whether through personal faith or participation in a religious community, spirituality often serves as a source of strength for families navigating the challenges of rare diseases.

Faith-Based Support

1. **Religious Communities**: Many families find hope and support through their religious communities, where they can share their struggles, receive prayers, and connect with others who understand the power of faith in times of difficulty. Religious institutions often offer both spiritual guidance and practical support,

helping families cope with their emotional and physical burdens.

2. **Prayer and Meditation**: For those who rely on faith, prayer and meditation offer a sense of peace and connection to something greater than themselves. These practices can help caregivers find hope in difficult situations, trusting that there is a purpose to their journey or that they are not alone in their struggles.

3. **Finding Meaning Through Faith**: Faith can also help families find meaning in their caregiving journey. Many parents express that their spirituality helps them understand their child's life as part of a greater plan, providing comfort even when faced with uncertainty or grief.

Hope is not a passive emotion but an active, transformative force that empowers families to navigate the challenges of rare diseases with resilience, perseverance, and courage. It sustains parents and caregivers through uncertainty, grief, and the many obstacles that arise, helping them focus on achievable goals and maintain faith in future possibilities.

Whether it comes from medical advocacy, community support, small victories in daily life, or deeply held spiritual beliefs, hope drives caregivers to seek the best possible outcomes for their children. It helps families to remain engaged in the fight for better treatments, to continue pursuing new opportunities, and to appreciate moments of joy even in the most difficult times.

Ultimately, hope is a powerful tool for survival and growth. It encourages families to keep striving, to remain connected with others, and to believe that despite the difficulties, a meaningful and fulfilling life is possible for both them and their children.

# CHAPTER 12: SUPPORTING THE SIBLINGS—ACKNOWLEDGING THE UNIQUE CHALLENGES AND NEEDS OF BROTHERS AND SISTERS

When a family is navigating the complexities of a child with a rare disease, it's easy for siblings to feel overshadowed. The needs of the affected child often take precedence, leaving siblings to manage their emotions in the background. These brothers and sisters may struggle with guilt, fear, jealousy, or even feelings of neglect, while also developing resilience, empathy, and a strong bond with their family. This chapter delves into the unique experiences of siblings, offering insight into their emotional challenges and practical strategies for parents to ensure that these siblings are supported and valued in their roles within the family.

## The Emotional and Psychological Impact on Siblings

Siblings of children with rare diseases often experience a wide range of emotions, many of which can go unnoticed. While they may understand the special care that their brother or sister needs, the imbalance in attention can lead to emotional distress. Below are the primary emotional and psychological responses common among siblings.

Feelings of Guilt and Confusion

1. **Survivor's Guilt**: Healthy siblings might feel guilty for not having the rare condition, questioning why they

were spared while their sibling has to endure significant hardships. This feeling, known as **survivor's guilt**, can manifest as self-blame or the belief that they don't deserve attention or praise because their sibling is "suffering more."

2. **Confusion About the Disease**: Especially for younger children, understanding a rare condition can be confusing. They may not grasp the full implications of their sibling's illness, leading to mixed feelings of fear and helplessness. Providing age-appropriate explanations can help demystify the situation and alleviate some of the confusion siblings feel.

Jealousy and Resentment

1. **Competing for Attention**: It's not uncommon for siblings to feel left out when the focus of family life revolves around medical appointments, treatments, and special accommodations for their sibling. This can lead to feelings of jealousy, even though the sibling may understand the necessity of the care. Without attention and validation, this jealousy can fester into resentment, making siblings feel emotionally isolated.

2. **Unfulfilled Needs**: Siblings may downplay their own needs or achievements because they don't want to add to their parents' already full plate. They might feel that their accomplishments, such as good grades or sports achievements, aren't as important compared to their sibling's medical struggles. This can contribute to a sense of neglect or frustration.

### Fear and Anxiety

The health of their sibling may be a source of constant worry for the healthy child. Whether the condition is life-threatening or manageable, uncertainty about the future can lead to chronic anxiety. Healthy siblings may worry about losing their sibling, witnessing medical emergencies, or dealing with the emotional strain on their parents. This fear can result in physical symptoms like stomach aches, sleep issues, or difficulty concentrating in school.

## Supporting Siblings' Emotional Resilience

Building emotional resilience in siblings is essential for helping them cope with the unique challenges they face. Emotional resilience allows siblings to process their feelings in healthy ways, maintain their own identity, and continue to feel connected to their family despite the demands placed on them by their sibling's condition.

Open Communication and Emotional Validation

1. **Encouraging Open Dialogue**: Creating a safe environment where siblings feel comfortable expressing their emotions is vital. Parents should encourage their children to talk about how they feel, even if those feelings are difficult. By acknowledging emotions such as frustration, jealousy, or sadness, parents can help siblings process these feelings and reduce any sense of guilt for having them.

2. **Providing Age-Appropriate Explanations**: Depending on their age and emotional development, siblings need different levels of information about their brother or sister's condition. Simplifying medical explanations for younger children while providing more detailed information to older siblings can reduce feelings of confusion and fear. Being transparent about the condition's impact also helps them understand why their sibling receives more attention at certain times.

3. **Validating Their Feelings**: It's important to let siblings know that their emotions are valid, whether it's sadness, jealousy, or guilt. Reassuring them that these feelings are natural and providing an outlet for them can prevent long-term emotional distress.

Encouraging Independence and Identity Development

1. **Fostering Individual Interests**: To help siblings develop their own sense of identity, parents can encourage them to pursue activities that allow them to shine, whether it's through sports, music, art, or academics. This helps siblings feel valued for who they are as individuals, rather than feeling like they are always in the shadow of their sibling's needs.

2. **Celebrating Siblings' Achievements**: Parents should make an effort to celebrate their other children's milestones and achievements. Even small gestures, such as attending a school play or celebrating good grades, can go a long way in helping siblings feel appreciated and seen. Acknowledging their successes can prevent feelings of neglect and ensure that they feel valued within the family.

### Creating Special Time for Siblings

Finding time for one-on-one interaction with siblings is crucial for strengthening family bonds. Even brief moments of individual attention can help siblings feel emotionally supported and reduce any feelings of being left out.

One-on-One Time with Parents

1. **Daily Check-ins**: Simple daily interactions, such as a conversation at breakfast or a few minutes before bed, can provide siblings with the opportunity to express

concerns or discuss their own lives. These check-ins offer a consistent reminder that their feelings and experiences are important.

2. **Special Outings**: Setting aside time for special outings with each sibling—whether it's a trip to the park, a movie night, or a visit to their favorite restaurant —can provide them with a break from the family's caregiving environment and give them undivided parental attention.

### Resources and Support for Siblings

Fortunately, many resources are available for siblings of children with rare diseases. These resources provide emotional and social support, helping siblings process their feelings and connect with others in similar situations.

Support Groups and Programs

1. **SuperSibs!**: A program under **Alex's Lemonade Stand Foundation**, **SuperSibs!** provides emotional support, online resources, and personalized encouragement for siblings of children with serious illnesses. Their goal is to help siblings feel valued and emotionally supported during their sibling's treatment.

2. **Sibshops (Sibling Support Project)**: **Sibshops** are workshops designed specifically for siblings of children with special needs, providing a space for siblings to meet others with similar experiences. These workshops focus on fun activities, peer support, and skill-building, allowing siblings to express their emotions and feel validated.

3. **Camp Sunshine**: **Camp Sunshine** offers family retreats and programs designed for families of children with life-threatening illnesses. They provide specific programs and activities for siblings, giving them the opportunity

to connect with others who understand their unique situation while also enjoying recreational activities.

## The Long-Term Effects on Siblings

While siblings face emotional challenges during childhood, they also develop valuable life skills that contribute to personal growth and empathy as adults. Many siblings of children with rare diseases develop a heightened sense of compassion, resilience, and emotional maturity that stays with them throughout their lives.

## Developing Empathy and Compassion

Growing up with a sibling who has a rare disease often fosters a deep sense of empathy and compassion. Siblings who have experienced the complexities of caregiving and health challenges tend to be more understanding of others' struggles. This increased empathy can lead to stronger relationships with friends, partners, and future colleagues.

## Building Resilience and Problem-Solving Skills

Siblings who experience the ups and downs of living with a rare disease in the family often develop strong problem-solving skills and resilience. They learn how to adapt to difficult situations, manage stress, and support others emotionally. These skills can serve them well into adulthood, influencing how they handle personal and professional challenges.

## Strengthening Family Bonds

Despite the challenges they face, many siblings develop strong, enduring bonds with their brother or sister with a rare disease. These relationships can become a source of comfort and strength throughout their lives, as the shared experience of managing a rare disease can create deep familial connections that transcend the hardships.

Supporting the siblings of children with rare diseases requires attention, understanding, and active effort from parents. By acknowledging their emotional needs, providing open communication, and ensuring they have opportunities to develop their own identities, families can help siblings thrive, even in the face of the challenges posed by a rare disease diagnosis.

With access to support groups, peer networks, and positive family dynamics, siblings can grow up feeling valued, emotionally secure, and connected to their family, enabling them to develop into empathetic, resilient adults who cherish the bonds they've formed during childhood.

# CHAPTER 13: NAVIGATING RELATIONSHIPS—MAINTAINING STRONG CONNECTIONS AMIDST CAREGIVING CHALLENGES

The impact of caring for a child with a rare disease is not limited to the medical and emotional needs of the child—it also profoundly affects family dynamics and relationships. Whether between parents, siblings, extended family members, or close friends, the added stress, time commitments, and emotional strain can lead to tension, misunderstanding, and distance in relationships. This chapter delves into the challenges that caregiving brings to relationships and offers practical strategies for maintaining healthy, supportive connections with partners, family, and friends.

## The Impact of Caregiving on Relationships

Caregiving is a demanding responsibility that often reconfigures the family structure and puts pressure on personal relationships. The complexities of managing a child's rare disease—including medical appointments, therapies, and day-to-day care—can create feelings of frustration, isolation, or resentment, particularly if the caregiving duties are unbalanced or misunderstood by others.

Changes in Marital and Partner Relationships

1. Increased Stress: The demands of caregiving often create stress in marital or partner relationships. Couples may experience conflicts over how to manage the child's care, finances, or household responsibilities. Additionally,

stress levels may increase if one partner feels that they are shouldering a disproportionate amount of the caregiving burden. Over time, this can erode the connection between partners.

2. Loss of Intimacy: The constant focus on the child's medical needs often leaves little time for partners to nurture their relationship. Many couples report a decrease in emotional and physical intimacy as their time and energy are diverted toward caregiving. This can lead to feelings of disconnection and loneliness within the relationship.

3. Differing Coping Mechanisms: Partners may cope with the stress of caregiving in different ways, leading to misunderstandings. One partner may prefer to talk openly about their worries, while the other might focus on practical solutions or avoid the subject altogether. Without open communication, these differences can create tension and emotional distance.

The Impact on Sibling Relationships

1. Feelings of Neglect: Siblings of children with rare diseases often feel neglected as the majority of their parents' attention is focused on the child with medical needs. This can lead to resentment, jealousy, or emotional withdrawal. Parents must balance their time to ensure that all children in the family feel valued and supported.

2. Overcompensation: In some cases, siblings may feel the need to overcompensate by excelling in school, sports, or other activities in an effort to gain their parents' attention. Alternatively, they may take on additional caregiving responsibilities, which can lead to feelings of guilt or burden. It's important for parents to recognize these dynamics and provide support to siblings as well.

Extended Family Dynamics

1. Lack of Understanding: Extended family members, such as grandparents, aunts, and uncles, may not fully understand the complexities of caring for a child with a rare disease. This lack of understanding can lead to hurtful comments or unsolicited advice, which can strain relationships. Caregivers often feel isolated or unsupported when family members fail to grasp the extent of their challenges.

2. Balancing Expectations: Caregivers may feel pressure from extended family members to maintain certain traditions or social obligations, even when those commitments become overwhelming due to their caregiving responsibilities. Managing these expectations can cause stress and tension within the family.

## Strengthening Marital and Partner Relationships

Despite the challenges caregiving presents, many couples find that it also brings opportunities for growth and deepens their bond. By prioritizing communication, sharing responsibilities, and making time for each other, couples can strengthen their relationship and work together to navigate the complexities of caregiving.

Prioritizing Communication

1. Open, Honest Conversations: Couples need to communicate openly about their feelings, concerns, and frustrations. Avoiding difficult conversations can lead to resentment or misunderstandings. By creating a safe space for honest dialogue, partners can work through their challenges and strengthen their emotional connection.

2. Regular Check-Ins: Setting aside time for regular check-ins—whether it's a daily conversation or a weekly meeting—can help couples stay connected and address any concerns before they escalate. During these check-ins, partners can discuss both practical matters (such as caregiving schedules) and emotional needs.

## Sharing Responsibilities

1. Delegating Tasks: To avoid burnout, it's essential for partners to share caregiving duties. This can include dividing up medical appointments, therapy sessions, or household chores. If one partner is the primary caregiver, the other can take on additional responsibilities to ease the caregiving burden.

2. Planning for Respite Time: Couples should prioritize respite time, both individually and together. Scheduling time for self-care or couple activities—even if it's as simple as a quiet dinner or a walk—can help partners reconnect and recharge. Respite care services or help from extended family can provide the necessary support to make this time possible.

## Rebuilding Intimacy

1. Small Gestures of Affection: Intimacy doesn't always require grand gestures. Small acts of affection—such as holding hands, sharing a cup of coffee, or sending a thoughtful text—can help maintain an emotional connection during stressful times.

2. Couples Therapy: For couples who are struggling to navigate the emotional toll of caregiving, couples therapy can be a valuable resource. A therapist can help partners improve communication, resolve conflicts, and rebuild emotional and physical intimacy.

### Engaging Extended Family and Friends

Maintaining strong relationships with extended family and friends can provide much-needed emotional support for caregivers. However, it's important to set clear boundaries and communicate effectively to ensure these relationships remain positive and supportive.

Educating Family and Friends

1. Providing Information About the Condition: Many family members and friends may not fully understand the complexities of the child's rare disease. Sharing educational materials or having open discussions about the child's condition can help increase understanding and reduce misunderstandings.

2. Setting Boundaries: Caregivers often need to set boundaries with family members who offer unsolicited advice or have unrealistic expectations. Politely but firmly setting these boundaries ensures that caregivers can focus on their child's needs without feeling overwhelmed by outside pressures.

Involving Family and Friends in Caregiving

1. Asking for Practical Help: Many extended family members and friends want to help but don't know how. Caregivers can ask for specific support, such as running errands, preparing meals, or providing occasional childcare. This can ease the caregiving burden and strengthen family bonds.

2. Hosting Family Events at Home: If attending family events becomes difficult due to caregiving responsibilities, inviting family members to your home can help maintain connections. Hosting small, low-

key gatherings allows caregivers to participate in social activities without the stress of travel.

# CONCLUSION: THRIVING TOGETHER—A JOURNEY OF HOPE, RESILIENCE, AND LOVE

As you come to the end of this book, it's important to reflect on the remarkable journey you've undertaken as a parent or caregiver of a child with a rare disease. This path is filled with challenges—medical complexities, emotional highs and lows, and moments of uncertainty. But it's also a journey marked by love, resilience, and a deep sense of purpose.

Throughout these pages, we've explored many aspects of caregiving: from advocating for your child's medical and educational needs to managing the emotional and financial burdens that can sometimes feel overwhelming. We've addressed the importance of self-care, the power of community, and the need to plan for the future to ensure that your child has a life filled with support and dignity.

However, what truly lies at the heart of this journey is love—the kind of unconditional love that drives parents and caregivers to push through the hardest days and find joy in the smallest victories. This love not only binds families together but also serves as the foundation of hope, sustaining you through the most difficult moments. It is this love that empowers you to advocate fiercely, to seek out the best care, and to keep searching for answers, even when the path ahead seems uncertain.

**You Are Not Alone**

One of the most isolating aspects of caring for a child with a rare disease is the feeling that no one truly understands what you are going through. But as we've emphasized throughout this book, you are not alone. There are countless families navigating similar challenges, and there are communities of support ready to lift you up when the weight feels too heavy. Whether through local support groups, online communities, or national advocacy organizations, you have a network of people who understand the unique journey you're on.

While the medical appointments, therapies, and educational planning can feel all-consuming, don't forget the importance of connection. Building and maintaining relationships with others —whether with family, friends, or fellow caregivers—will help sustain you. The strength and resilience you cultivate will not only benefit your child but also enrich your own life in ways you might not yet fully realize.

**Resilience Through Hope**

Resilience is not something that happens overnight. It's built over time through experience, reflection, and the choices we make every day to persevere despite the challenges. As parents and caregivers, you are constantly navigating the unknown, but with every step forward, you build a deeper well of resilience. Each day is an opportunity to learn, grow, and adapt to new circumstances, but above all, it's a chance to cultivate hope.

Hope is what fuels progress. It's what inspires families to seek new treatments, fight for their child's rights, and envision a future filled with possibilities. Even in the face of medical uncertainties or difficult diagnoses, hope gives you the strength to keep going. It reminds you that no matter how complex the journey may be, there are always resources, communities, and individuals who are working toward the same goal—helping your child live their best life.

## Thriving Together

Caregiving for a child with a rare disease is not just about survival; it's about thriving together as a family. It's about finding moments of joy amid the challenges, creating lasting memories, and forging bonds that grow stronger through shared experiences. While the road may be difficult, it's important to remember that your family's love and resilience are powerful forces. Together, you will find a way not only to manage the day-to-day demands but also to celebrate the unique and beautiful journey you are on.

As you move forward, continue to advocate, continue to care for yourself, and continue to foster a sense of community around you. Every small step forward, every act of love, and every moment of care you provide for your child is a testament to your strength. While the challenges will persist, so will the love, the hope, and the support that surround you.

This book is not the end of your journey—it's a companion that will be with you as you continue to navigate the complex and rewarding path of caring for a child with a rare disease. You are not alone, and together, you and your family will thrive.

# REFERENCES AND RESOURCES

To support your journey, here are several key resources mentioned throughout the book. These organizations, tools, and services offer invaluable guidance, assistance, and community support for families caring for a child with a rare disease.

Advocacy and Support Organizations

1. Global Genes
   A leading global organization providing resources, advocacy, and support for families affected by rare diseases.
   Website: globalgenes.org

2. National Organization for Rare Disorders (NORD)
   NORD offers a comprehensive list of rare diseases, patient assistance programs, and advocacy support for families navigating the complexities of a rare disease diagnosis.
   Website: rarediseases.org

3. The Mighty
   An online community where parents and caregivers can share their stories, find support, and connect with others facing similar challenges.
   Website: themighty.com

4. RareConnect
   A platform that connects rare disease patients and their families through discussion forums, personal stories, and community engagement.
   Website: rareconnect.org

Financial Assistance Programs

1.  Patient Access Network Foundation
    Offers co-pay assistance for prescription medications
    and other medical costs.
    Website: panfoundation.org

2.  UnitedHealthcare Children's Foundation
    Provides medical grants to cover health-related services
    not covered by insurance, such as therapies, surgeries,
    and equipment.
    Website: uhccf.org

3.  NORD's RareCare® Patient Assistance Program
    Offers financial assistance for medications, travel,
    and treatment-related costs for individuals with rare
    diseases.
    Website: rarediseases.org/assistance-programs

Medical Resources

1.  ClinicalTrials.gov
    A database of clinical trials, providing up-to-date
    information on research studies, new treatments, and
    therapies for rare diseases.
    Website: clinicaltrials.gov

2.  National Institutes of Health (NIH) Genetic and Rare
    Diseases (GARD) Information Center
    Provides comprehensive information on rare diseases,
    including treatment options and ongoing research
    efforts.
    Website: rarediseases.info.nih.gov

Educational Resources

1.  Wrightslaw
    A leading resource for information on special education

law and advocacy for children with disabilities, including guidance on IEPs and 504 Plans.
Website: wrightslaw.com

2. The Sibling Support Project
Provides workshops, support, and resources for the siblings of children with disabilities and rare diseases.
Website: siblingsupport.org

Mental Health and Caregiver Support

1. ARCH National Respite Network
Helps connect families with respite care services, allowing caregivers time to rest and recharge.
Website: archrespite.org

2. The Compassionate Friends
Offers support for parents grieving the loss of a child, with both local and online communities for emotional support.
Website: compassionatefriends.org

These resources are here to support you in all areas of caregiving—whether you need emotional support, financial assistance, or guidance on navigating the healthcare and educational systems. Remember, this journey is shared, and there is a vast network of people, organizations, and tools available to help you every step of the way.

# COMMUNITY RESPONDERS LLC

337 N Mesa Drive #102
Mesa Arizona 85201

480.521.1107

www.comrestraining.com

www.ingramcontent.com/pod-product-compliance
Lightning Source LLC
Chambersburg PA
CBHW071039250726
48653CB00005B/1898